The Study Skills Handbook for Nutritionists and Dietitians

The Study Skills Handbook for Nutritionists and Dietitians

Sue Reeves and Yvonne Jeanes

Open University Press

Open University Press
McGraw-Hill Education
8th Floor, 338 Euston Road
London
England
NW1 3BH

email: enquiries@openup.co.uk
world wide web: www.openup.co.uk

and Two Penn Plaza, New York, NY 10121-2289, USA

First edition published 2022

A catalogue record of this book is available from the British Library

Commissioning Editor: Sam Crowe
Associate Editor: Beth Summers
Content Product Manager: Ali Davis
Head of Portfolio Marketing: Bryony Waters

ISBN-13: 9780335250455
ISBN-10: 0335250459
eISBN: 9780335250462

Library of Congress Cataloging-in-Publication Data
CIP data applied for

Typeset by Transforma Pvt. Ltd., Chennai, India

Praise page

"*This book contains everything that students of nutrition or dietetics may require to improve their study skills, from essay writing and critical appraisal to how to display data, prepare a presentation and design an academic poster. Uniquely, the examples and exercises are all specific to our fascinating discipline. Using their extensive experience of university teaching as well as pedagogic theory, the authors have created an essential compendium to support students throughout their learning journey; from day 1 of their degree up to their first steps into a career in nutrition and dietetics.*"

Professor Kevin Whelan, Head of Department of Nutritional Sciences, King's College London

"*This study guide has been produced by two well respected nutrition professionals. It is an extremely helpful aid for all those studying nutrition or dietetics, providing the reader with a plethora of practical information, tips, and advice to support not only their studies, but also their journey to becoming a Registered Nutritionist or Dietitian. I can see this being a valuable text on many a nutrition professional's bookcase, mine included.*"

Dr Glenys Jones RNutr, Deputy Chief Executive, Association for Nutrition

"'*The Study Skills Handbook for Nutritionists and Dietitians*' *by Dr Sue Reeves and Dr Yvonne Jeanes is a* <u>must</u> *read for all current and future Nutritionists and Dietitians – both Academics and Students alike. It is hugely insightful; comprehensively written and richly resourced. The authors are to be commended for covering aspects for both Nutritionists and Dietitians. It is an outstanding Handbook and written to the highest of standards. I recommend it most highly.*"

Professor Susan Lanham-New, Head of the Nutritional Sciences Department & Professor of Human Nutrition, University of Surrey

"*This book is a valuable resource for students studying to become either a Registered Nutritionist or Dietitian, and which contains a variety of exciting topics to support both students' study skills but also their personal and professional development. It has been written by esteemed and experienced colleagues with long experience in educating future nutrition professionals. This textbook not only contains everything that students need to become successful nutritionists and dietitians, but it can also serve as a tool for Nutrition and Dietetics curriculum design."*

Dr Katerina Vafeiadou RNutr, Senior Lecturer in
Nutrition & Dietetics, University of Hertfordshire

"It was a delight to review this book. It provides all the study skills required for dietetics and nutrition students in one place. This book covers what students need from foundation year to postgraduate study. It is a comprehensive overview on how to be able to deliver evidence-based, service-user centred dietetic care and innovative public health nutrition initiatives across a range of client groups and working environments."

Dr Samireh Jorfi, Senior Lecturer, London Metropolitan University

Contents

Acknowledgements

We would like to thank the Nutrition team at the University of Roehampton who are always so supportive and full of good ideas; Astrid Hauge-Evans, Adele Costabile, Giulia Corona, Michael Patterson, Patrick Brady and Steven Trangmar.

We thank all our past students who have helped inform our teaching and learning practices. We listened and reflected on how we can develop to help future students improve their experience and achievements during their degrees and as they start their careers culminating in this book.

Thanks also to Sam Crowe, Beth Summers, and Ali Davis from Open University Press and McGraw Hill Education for guiding us so smoothly through the whole book writing process.

Finally our families for all their support and encouragement.

Author biography

Dr Sue Reeves is the Head of Undergraduate Studies and Student Experience in the School of Life Sciences and Health Sciences at the University of Roehampton. She has taught nutrition for over 20 years, has won teaching excellence awards, has been an external examiner, and is a Senior Fellow of the Higher Education Academy. She is a Registered Nutritionist and a Fellow of the Association for Nutrition, where she is also a CPD assessor and Regional Representative. Her published research includes many aspects of nutrition including the role of diet in obesity, coeliac disease, and healthy and sustainable restaurants. Sue is part of the international Toybox Malaysia team that has been awarded two Medical Research Council grants for projects to improve healthy energy balance and obesity related behaviours among pre-schoolers in Malaysia, and is an advisor on degree programmes in Malaysia and Singapore.

Dr Yvonne Jeanes is a registered dietitian with current clinical, teaching and research experience. She is the Head of Postgraduate Taught Provision within the School of Life and Health Sciences at the University of Roehampton and is a Senior Fellow of the Higher Education Academy. She has been an external examiner for BSc Nutrition and Dietetic programmes and has taught undergraduates and postgraduate healthcare professionals for over 15 years. Dr Jeanes is the Research and Policy lead for the British Dietetic Association Gastroenterology Specialist Group. Her research focuses on dietetic outcomes, nutritional adequacy and practicalities of living gluten free with coeliac disease. She has lead studies that have informed UK government policy and is currently co leading two national projects in coeliac disease and irritable bowel syndrome.

Part A

1 Introduction

Overview and outline

Starting university is an exciting time but it is only natural that you might be a little nervous and not entirely sure what is expected of you academically. We wrote this book with the aim of helping you identify and develop the study skills you need to support your learning, do well in class and with assessments. We want you to do well on your chosen course and make the most of all the opportunities you have in front of you whilst studying for your degree and beyond.

This book was initially created for students who are studying to be an Associate Registered Nutritionist or a Dietitian; however, we hope students on other courses will also find much of this information relevant to them as well. Whether you are a fresher, or about to start a postgraduate programme, we wanted to ensure you had a handbook that could provide all the study skills you need in one place. If you are preparing to start a new course you might want to read this book all the way through from start to finish. However, you may prefer to use this book to dip in and out whenever you need to brush up on particular skills. Either way, we hope this book covers everything you need from foundation year or first year undergraduate to postgraduate study, as well as offering some tips for preparing for the workplace.

We both teach at a university and recognise that the transition to higher education can be challenging for some students, and that not all students have confidence in their own academic skills. We planned this book with the aim of providing you with the knowledge and skills to empower you to take control of your learning, boost your confidence, be prepared for new challenges and help you succeed at university. We would also like to encourage you to try to be an active learner who can reflect on your academic and professional development as you begin to plan your career ahead as an Associate Registered Nutritionist or a Dietitian.

Outline of the book

Each chapter of the book covers different areas of academic study but the common thread that runs through the entire book, and what links each chapter, is the focus on the skills required to be an Associate Registered Nutritionist or a Dietitian.

The book is divided into two sections: Part A focuses on more traditional study skills, using nutrition and dietetic examples, and Part B is aimed at preparing you for a career post-graduation.

Part A includes the following skills:

- Scientific writing including literature reviews, essays and reports
- Collecting and presenting data
- Referencing
- Group work
- Oral presentations
- Poster presentations
- How to work online
- Preparing for exams
- Making the most of feedback

Part B will outline what it means to be not just a graduate, but also an Associate Registered Nutritionist or a Dietitian. This includes work that might require consultations for individuals or groups, and ensuring you maintain your continuing professional development (CPD).

Each chapter starts with an overview and outline section to explain the key features that will be covered. Information is presented in a similar style to what we give to our students in module guides and lectures. Nutrition and dietetic examples have been used throughout so you can see how they might be applied to your work and your future career. We have also provided summaries at the end of each chapter and suggested further reading as well as some questions to help you contemplate the topics covered as you start to develop reflective practice.

Why do you need study skills?

We know study skills might not seem the most exciting topic; you might even think that you learnt all this at school. We also understand that you might want to jump straight into the content of your degree and start designing menus and analysing diets. However, study skills are essential for all your studies and will underpin every piece of work you do. Furthermore, now you are at university it is anticipated that you will develop these skills further and to a higher standard. Such skills take time to develop: they will grow and progress during your time at university. If you keep your mind open to learning and practising them, you will be rewarded. Having these skills will bring you confidence and put you more in control. You can focus on the exciting content knowing you have the basics in hand. Even if you think you have all the study skills you need, there are bound to be certain assignments that will be new to you, and require you to use skills you have not used before, or require details that are easy to forget but which can affect your final grade. So take the time to continue to develop your skills even further. Moreover, all of these skills are transferable, which means you can put them on your CV and you will definitely use them in your next job.

Transition to university

We know starting university can be nerve wracking for some people, but never worry that you aren't good enough: you were accepted onto the course in the first place, so your lecturers certainly think you have what it takes.

You will most likely be assigned a tutor when you start university. This person might have different titles such as 'academic guidance tutor' or 'personal tutor' but essentially they offer the same support. Your tutor is often your first port of call should you have any questions. They will take an interest in your progress and will help you make the most of your time at university. They can provide advice for assessment, they may have revision tips, and they can help you understand your feedback. It's important that you communicate with your tutor so that they know what is happening; when you are offered meetings it is important you attend. Your tutor may not have the answer to everything, but they are sure to know who to put you in touch with if they can't help; they can act as a gatekeeper to signpost other university services. Make sure you play your part in keeping communication channels open with your tutor.

Studying at university is probably going to include much more independent learning than you might have experienced at school or college, and you will need to take responsibility for your own learning. Establish what works best for you and work in your own way. Through reflective practice (which we discuss in detail in Chapter 9) you can find out what your strengths and weaknesses are and then take responsibility for maintaining those strengths and working on your weaknesses.

Be an active learner

We want to encourage you to become an 'active learner'. Active learning puts the emphasis on how you learn not just what you learn and has been shown to be associated with positive outcomes including test marks and grades (Smith and Cardaciotto 2011). Your lecturers will consider this when planning their lectures and lessons to incorporate different activities to help keep you actively engaged such as:

- Quizzes
- Case studies

- Problem solving
- Lab work
- Presentations
- Discussions

You can make sure you take an active rather than passive approach to your learning too. Just listening to a lecture may not be the best way to learn and retain information. But making notes, annotating or illustrating them and testing yourself and applying your knowledge are great ways to understand the material and then retain what you have learnt. Find out what methods work best for you to keep yourself engaged and make progress with the taught material. Being an active learner is something you can continue even after you have graduated as you develop the mind set required to be a life-long learner.

Time management

Taking responsibility for your own learning will also require good time management skills. It might be useful to get a diary or some sort of planner. Work out when your lectures are but also ensure you plan time for independent study, any online required content such as recorded lectures, and time for working on assignments to ensure they can be submitted punctually. Remember to think about your other commitments and time for relaxation. Having a routine in place can help you keep on top of your work, be more productive and, most importantly, less stressed.

Critical thinking

A large part of your degree will involve critical thinking. This has been described as: '*the art of making clear, reasoned judgements based on interpreting, understanding, applying and synthesising evidence gathered from observation, reading and experimentation*' (Burns and Sinfield 2016).

Developing your critical thinking skills may take some work but it is very important to your achievements at university; with practice it will become second nature. In nutrition and dietetics, you will come across lots of different sources of information. Some of it may be anecdotal, some may be evidence based, but you need to be able to see the difference and able to make scientific judgements based on the quality and accuracy of the information you are presented with. In fact, Riis et al. (2019) have stated that fake news spreads further than factual news, particularly on social media, and this is especially true when it comes to nutrition information. We need to be ready to question the evidence base for such news and approach it in critical and perhaps even sceptical way. This does not mean you have to be critical of the opinions of others; instead, you need to question the information and the sources of that information with an open mind, as you develop your own ideas and learn to debate in a well-reasoned and informed way.

After you graduate

When you have just started at university, graduation can seem like a long way off. However, it is worth considering what you would like to do when you graduate so you can plan for this in advance. It might mean going to careers talks, getting work experience or a placement during the vacations, or completing relevant webinars to expand your knowledge in particular areas. It could involve attending a conference and networking with people who already have a career in the area in which you would like to work. Being an employable graduate is not only about having a degree; there are also certain skills that you are expected to have, including the study skills we describe in this book. It is these skills and qualities that will make you not only employable but also a valued colleague.

Summary

We want you to enjoy your time at university and hopefully this chapter has explained why study skills are important and how developing them can help your confidence and put you in control of your studies. We have also outlined the importance of being organised and being an active learner and critical thinker. Finally, when writing this book, we wanted to remind you why you chose and wanted to study to be an Associate Registered Nutritionist or a Dietitian in the first place. We know many of you, like us, are passionate about nutrition and dietetics, and we don't want you to lose sight of that as you plan your future career. We hope you learn lots from this book to help you excel but most importantly enjoy your studies.

Reflective questions

- Why did you choose to study Nutrition or Dietetics?
- What do you hope to achieve by the time you have completed your chosen programme?
- Are you ready to get started?

References

Burns, T. and Sinfield, S. (2016) *Essential Study Skills: The Complete Guide to Success at University*, 4th edn. London: SAGE, p94.

Riis J., McFadden, B.R. and Collins, K. (2019) Thinking critically about nutrition. *Today's Dietitian* 21: 36.

Smith, V.C. and Cardaciotto, L.A. (2011) Is active learning like broccoli? Student perceptions of active learning in large lecture classes, *Journal of the Scholarship of Teaching and Learning*, 11(1): 53–61.

2 Scientific writing

Overview and outline

You will rely heavily on your scientific writing skills whilst at university and they will be essential for many of your assessments. These are skills that you will also need later when you are in the workplace, so it makes sense to hone these skills now as you will make great use of them. In this chapter we will explore writing styles and different types of written work, including essays, literature reviews, reports and case studies, but we will also consider how to get started and get writing.

Introduction

Being able to communicate clearly in writing is an important skill to master since it is a key method for disseminating and sharing scientific findings. As Dietitians and Associate Registered Nutritionists, you will need to be able to keep accurate written records and to present your findings for others to read, additionally you will also need to review and summarise the scientific literature. Scientific writing may be slightly different from other forms of writing in that it is factual and formal; however, it should always be clear and concise. Scientific writing is a process that needs regular practice (Peterson et al. 2018), so try to find time in your schedule to sit down and focus on your writing.

Writing style

Scientific writing is usually rather impersonal and where possible we encourage the use of the passive voice, rather than the active voice, avoiding personal pronouns such as 'we', 'you' and 'I'. For example, if you were describing how you analysed some food diaries you might write:

I analysed the three-day food diaries...

However in the passive voice this could be written as:

The three-day food diaries were analysed...

This can take some getting used to, and in many cases your lecturers would prioritise writing clearly over using the passive voice, if this is something you really struggle with. But we can assure you it does get easier with practice. (Please note, however, we deliberately chose not to use the strictly formal scientific style for this book as we wanted to make it more personable.)

Science writing is usually quite cautious and tends not to make grand statements unless we are 100 per cent sure they are true. We use words and phrases like 'in general' or 'the results appear to show'. Particularly when talking about people, we must take care not to overgeneralise as there are often exceptions. However, the more exact you can be the better so if you can quantify a statement by including data (referenced of course) then please do, for example '88 per cent of women met the recommendations for …'.

Try to be neutral and objective when you consider the literature and put together your written arguments based on an accurate representation of the facts. You should also try to avoid rhetorical questions, i.e. questions where you don't expect an actual answer such as 'Want to get more fibre in your diet?' Although rhetorical style questions are common in magazine articles they are not usually used in scientific writing, which is generally a precise presentation of facts. So instead of writing 'Want to get more fibre in your diet?' you could write 'To increase the fibre content of the diet … '.

Your writing should be understandable, so don't over complicate things or use technical jargon when it is not necessary. Any scientific concepts or specialist terms always need to be explained clearly. Try to avoid unnecessary abbreviations and instead write the words in full; for example, 'isn't' should be written as 'is not'. If you are using acronyms try not to overdo them, as this can confound your message, and make sure you define them on first use, e.g. dietary induced thermogenesis (DIT).

Getting started and overcoming writer's block

Getting started is often the hardest part and looking at an empty piece of paper or screen can be quite off putting. For this reason, we say just write anything anywhere on the page. You can go back and edit, or even delete it later, but getting something on the page is a good start. Writing key words or general brain storming all help to fill the page and get you started. You could even just put a scribble on the page if that helped you avoid blank page syndrome! Writing down paragraph headings, or the main points you want to make, can also help, and then you can go back and begin to expand on them.

Another good tip if you struggle to start writing, is to talk about it. You could tell a friend or even talk to yourself about what you want to write, record it on your phone and transcribe that onto paper. You can then edit and add more details as required.

You don't have to start at the beginning, you can start anywhere, so if you already have the information you need for a later paragraph – why not write that one first? Write the bits you are more confident with and then go back and fill in the other parts when you are further along. If you get stuck mid-sentence don't worry just leave a space or add some xxxxx's; keep going and come back to that point later.

Avoid procrastinating and putting it off for another day: if you leave yourself too little time this will only add to your worries. Make a plan, or a timetable, and try to stick to it. You could even go back and look at pieces you have written before, as proof to yourself that you can do this.

Essays

Essays are a common type of assessment at university, so it is very likely that you will need to write one at some point. Not only will this assess your knowledge and understanding of the subject, but your research, writing and organisational skills too.

Understanding the title

The first thing you need to do is consider the title of the essay. Take your time and make sure you really understand it. You should read the title several times and really pick it apart and analyse what it means.

First, pick out the key subject words, those that tell you what the essay is about. You should also look for the command words. These indicate what you are expected to do. Some examples of common command words are shown in Table 2.1.

Also, check your essay title to see if there are any particular instructions to follow. This might include ensuring you include certain points in your essay or perhaps you are instructed to use examples in your answer.

Activity

Look at the two essay titles below. Can you identify the key words, the command words and if there are any instructions?

1 Compare and contrast Kwashiorkor and Marasmus.
2 Explain the importance of post-exercise nutrition and give examples of recovery strategies for named sports.

Check the word limits

Word limits will vary, so make sure you check this before starting. You should aim to get as close as possible to the word limit, though many universities will accept 10 per cent above or below this limit. The word limit will also give you an indication of how much detail you need to go into. If you think you have finished but your essay is only 1000 words when your word limit is 2000, you know you need to provide a lot more detail and you may even need to do some more research. If you have gone over your word limit, have you gone off track

Table 2.1 Common command words in essay titles

Command word	Meaning
Describe	Give a description of the topic (*this is more likely to be used for foundation or first year work*)
Outline	Identify the main points
State	Describe precisely and clearly
Compare	Show the similarities and differences
Explain	Clarify why something happens or why it may occur
Examine	Look in detail
Define	Describe what is meant by
Discuss	Consider the arguments for and against
Contrast	Compare the differences between
Evaluate	Assess the importance
Analyse	Breakdown and examine the parts
Critically evaluate	Consider the strengths and weakness and make an assessment (*more likely to be used for third year or postgraduate work*)

and included less relevant information or have you 'waffled' perhaps? Either way, aim to get as close as you can to the required number of words you have been given.

Make a plan

It is certainly worth making an essay plan. This could be a visual plan, such as a spider diagram where you jot down ideas all over the page, or something more linear, where perhaps you list the paragraph headings you intend to use; you can always delete these headings later.

The box below presents an example of a linear style of plan for an essay.

Example of an essay plan: linear style

Title: *Using named examples, describe the pros and cons of different methods of dietary analysis that need to be considered when deciding which is the most appropriate method for particular population groups (2000 words)*
Introduction *~200 words*

Main body

Each paragraph considers the pros & cons and suitability for different population groups

1 *Food diaries* *~300 words*
2 *Food frequency questionnaire (FFQ)* *~300 words*
3 *Recall* *~300 words*
4 *Diet history* *~300 words*
5 *Emerging technologies* *~300 words*

Conclusion *including summary ~300 words*
References

Information gathering

Before you get started on the writing you will need to research the topic of the essay. Lecture notes are a good place to start, followed by recommended textbooks and journal papers; these will also be essential as you will want to ensure you are using appropriate sources. As you progress through your degree and certainly for postgraduate study online database search for journal review and original articles are particularly important. Suggested reading for comprehensive literature searching is Chapter 4 of Hickson (2018). Take care to stay focused; don't get side-tracked and do stick to your plan.

Start by jotting down all your ideas and making notes from your research; be selective and only make notes on information you can use in your essay. Take time to read and assimilate the information from different sources before writing it down in your own words. Ensure you also keep a note of the source of any materials as this will save a lot of time later, should you need to go back to the original material to check anything, and also for referencing purposes.

Then gather all the information you have. Try to organise it so that you group similar pieces of information together; you don't want to put information on the same topic in different places. Similarly, take care not to repeat the same information in slightly different ways.

Building your essay: sentences and paragraphs

Each sentence should be complete and make sense. Think about your choice of words to make each sentence as precise as possible. Your essay should be organised into paragraphs, which usually should be more than one sentence long.

Each paragraph would normally have a central theme and you should always start a new paragraph for a new point or theme. The PEEL method is a popular framework for structuring paragraphs that you may have come across. PEEL is an acronym that stands for:

Point – establish the point you are trying to make
Evidence – provide an example of something that proves your point

Evaluate – consider the evidence and why this point supports your argument
Link – the last sentence should sum up that paragraph and link back to the
   original point, or link to the next paragraph.

You could perhaps start with the easiest points that you want to include in
your essay and take it one paragraph at a time. Think about the order of each
paragraph. You can move paragraphs around if you need, so that they flow
from one to another in a logical manner, and to give your essay structure.

Essay structure

Essays may not have a formal structure in the way a report does (see later in
this chapter); however, they are usually organised into the following sections:

- Introduction
- Main body
- Conclusion
- References

The introduction always relates strictly to the essay title, sets the scene
and lays out what the reader might expect. It will probably be only one or two
paragraphs long.

The main body of the essay is where you present the key information, the
arguments for and against, and where you add all the details. This can be sub-
divided into different paragraphs, organised in a logical and sequential way
(see the PEEL method above). By all means use paragraph headings if this
helps you organise your material. The facts you present should be referenced
so that each point you make is supported by evidence. You may use figures or
tables in an essay if you need to, but only do this if the information is key and
would really enhance your essay (not just to fill up space), Ensure you refer to
each figure or table in the text plus give each a title and reference.

The conclusion draws all your points together and relates this information
back to the original question or the title of the essay. This section is usually
only one paragraph long.

First draft

Don't worry too much about your first draft: focus on getting words onto the
page. You know you can improve things when you redraft and proofread later.
But try to get your main points down and check your argument is clear. Table
2.2 presents some of the key differences between strong and weak essays. See
how your essay compares with this: are there changes you can make that will
make your essay stronger?

Re-drafting and fine tuning

You may need to write several drafts before you are happy. Think about cutting
and pasting whatever you need so that the essay flows; each point leading on

Table 2.2   Differences between strong and weak essays

A strong essay will:	A weak essay will:
Show clear understanding of the material	Show misunderstanding of the material
Be the correct style, structure and length	No structure, too short or too long
Have a logical argument	No clear argument
Show originality	Irrelevant content
Include critique	Largely descriptive
Use appropriate references, cited correctly	No references used

to the next. You might look more closely now at your use of language: is it as precise as it could be? You should also check the grammar and spelling; but don't rely solely on your computer's automated spelling and grammar checkers, as although they will highlight when a word is misspelt, they won't show you when you have used the wrong word. For example, think about 'loose' and 'lose' – both are spelt correctly but have very different meanings. Make sure that when you save each draft you label it clearly so you know which file to come back to and ensure you submit the correct copy.

For tips about writing essays in exam conditions look at Chapter 7.

Literature and critical reviews

The terms 'literature review' and 'critical review' are often used interchangeably. In fact you could say that a literature review is a type of critical review. Critical reviews may review just one paper or they may include many papers; however, a literature review will always include many papers. The focus here will be on literature reviews.

Literature reviews aim to evaluate the published literature on a specific area of interest and are usually semi-structured, following this format.

They all start with an **introduction** to present the topic and set out what the literature review aims to cover. This section may also make clear how you are defining specific terms or key concepts that are central to your review.

Some but not all literature reviews have a **methods** section. A methods section in a literature review is likely to very briefly describe your search terms and your inclusion and exclusion criteria; e.g. 'all articles needed to be written in English and peer reviewed. *In vitro* and animal studies were excluded.' You can name the search engines you used, and the time frame you considered; e.g. 'PubMed and Science Direct were used to find all papers published between 1 January 2000 and 31 March 2022.'

Then there will be the **main body** of the text, where you describe and critique the studies you have read. You should try to collate the information from different sources, grouping similar papers together and showing how some research findings may have led to subsequent research. Compare and contrast different results and also the reasons for those differences as you evaluate the studies. Start a new paragraph for different parts of the argument or for different themes.

Finally, complete your review with a **conclusion** based on the literature you reviewed.

Annotated bibliography

An annotated bibliography is different from a literature review in that each paper included is described and reviewed in turn, so it is more like a list of key papers. Whereas literature reviews will try and collate and synthesise the research, annotated bibliographies will take each paper one at a time. Although you will need to describe the paper and the findings, you must also provide some critique or assessment of the paper too.

Report writing

As part of your programme, you are sure to be involved in some practical work such as doing experiments in the laboratory. This sort of work is usually written up as a formal scientific report where you can describe what you did, what results you got and what they mean. Reports usually have a standard structure and this is described below.

But before you get started, check your instructions. You may be asked to include specific data tables or graphs, and on rare occasions leave out certain sections.

Sections of a scientific report
  i. **Title** – You will probably be given this; however, if you need to come up with your own title, keep it concise but ensure it describes the report adequately. For example. 'Investigation into the protein content of organic and non-organic milk' is more descriptive than 'Proteins in milk'.
 ii. **Abstract** – This is a summary of the whole report and should include a brief summary of the purpose, what you did and what you found. Although it is the first paragraph someone will read, you might make this the last section you write, leaving it until you have all your information and know what your conclusion is.
iii. **Introduction** – This provides the rationale and sets the scene for the whole report. It describes what has been done before and gives the

essential background details. This will include a review of the literature which, depending on the length of the report, could be a brief summary of a few key references or an in-depth review if it is a large report. Any gaps in the literature and knowledge should be identified here. Introductions usually finish with the aim of the report.

iv. **Methods** – This is where you describe what was done. You should give step-by-step details about the protocol, the equipment used and the measurements made. Any specialist equipment should be named, and the manufacturer and location given, e.g. 'weighing scales (Seca, Birmingham)' likewise particular computer packages that were used, e.g. 'Dietplan 7 (Forestfield Software, Sussex)'. If your study included any human participants you need to state that ethical approval was given and by whom. You should also provide details about the software you used and statistical tests performed to analyse the data. This section should always be written strictly past tense. You may have been told that the methods section is like a recipe and should be reported in such a way that anyone could follow it. Whilst the level of detail required may be similar, please note that recipes are usually written in an active tense, e.g. 'mix the ingredients', whereas methods sections should be written in the past tense e.g. 'the ingredients were mixed'. Be as concise as possible without leaving out key details.

v. **Results** – What did you find? Use this section to present your data and remember you are just presenting your data here, not discussing it (that is for the next section). Include any appropriate graphs and tables. Avoid replicating the same data in two different ways, so if the data is presented most clearly in a table you don't need to add a graph just for the sake of it, and vice versa. All tables and graphs should be numbered and have a title, in order to stand alone. However, there must be explanatory text above or below the figures which relates to the tables and graphs and explains your findings in words. In most cases you should use the International System of Units (SI), e.g. height in metres (m) and weight in kilograms (kg). However, although we should present energy in kJ, it is still common in nutrition and dietetics to use kilocalories (kcal).

vi. **Discussion** – This is where you explain and interpret your findings and relate them to your original aims. Here you can highlight your thinking and understanding of the results and what they mean. It is often good to start with a summary of the results you found, before going on to discuss what they mean and how they compare to the results of previously published work. If your results are different to what you might have expected, try to consider why this may have occurred. Use references in this section to back up all your arguments and for the other studies you are comparing. Consider also, the limitations of your study, and what could be done differently to improve it.

vii. **Conclusion** – Summarise your findings and put them into context here. You shouldn't introduce any new points, instead this is where you close the report.

viii. References – Any references cited in the report should be listed here.

  ix. Appendices – Put here any raw data, calculations or additional information not central to the report, such as recipes or policy documents for example.

Case study

Case studies are a type of problem-based learning, and these usually reflect a true-to-life situation where you apply the theory to a practical situation. Case studies can be theoretical or real (perhaps part of a clinical placement). If the case study is based on a real patient, then you will need to ensure you have informed consent from both the patient and the lead clinician; most importantly, the case study must be anonymous – you should exclude the name and any identifiable descriptors to protect confidentiality.

Case studies are usually descriptive, written in the active tone of voice and are more personal. However, whilst case studies can provide an in-depth analysis of a real life situation, it should be recognised that they can be unique to the individual rather than generalised and therefore may not always be representative.

The layout of a case study can vary, and your university may even have a proforma for you to complete, so do check that first. However, most case studies will include some or all of the following sections:

* **Introduction** – where you can set out the background and establish the purpose of the case study.
* **Methods used** – this might include: anthropometry, biochemistry, clinical history, dietary intakes.
* **Results or findings** – you can include any data here.
* **Discussion and evaluation** – this may include your nutritional diagnosis and what this means. You may need to consider other circumstances and how they may impact any dietary treatment given.
* **Recommendations, Implementation, Monitoring** – this should be based on your findings, should be realistic, practical and include a time frame.
* **Conclusion** – summarise the outcomes of your case study.
* **References** – as before, list any references cited here.
* **Appendices** – include any raw data or additional information.

Written presentation

For all written work, do take some time to consider the presentation. Although it is the content that for the most part is the important thing, ensuring that your work looks neat and professional will certainly help give the reader a good impression. Consider the following.

- Are you using a clear font and is it the same font throughout the document?
- Is the point size big enough to read easily? Usually size 11 or 12 is best; leave anything bigger for titles.
- Are there clearly defined paragraphs?
- Are the margins justified to the left (so the edges of text on the left side of the page are straight)?
- Fully justified (where the edges are straight on both the left and right sides of the page) can look neat and tidy but can also result in strange gaps in the middle of lines, which can sometimes look a bit odd.
- Centred text should only be used for titles.
- Double line spacing usually looks better and is often preferred by lecturers for marking as there is more space to write comments.
- Generally you should avoid using CAPITAL letters, if you want something, like paragraph headings, to stand out – use **bold**.
- Don't forget to insert the page numbers, especially if it is a long piece of work.

Final checks

Remember to allow enough time to proofread your work carefully. Check you have answered the question or have met the aim, and consider your language, spelling and grammar. Take another look at the presentation too: could this be improved? You may need to edit your work several times before you get it right, and editing is all part of the craft of writing. Printing out your work to read might make it easier to spot small mistakes. Reading your work out loud can help too, so you can check that every sentence is complete and makes sense. It is always worth coming back to a piece of work the next day with fresh eyes; you will be amazed at the things you pick up that you hadn't previously noticed. However, if you are tinkering with the writing and starting to change words for the sake of it, or you are obsessing over a minor point, then it is time to stop the editing, submit the work and step away from the keyboard.

Summary

Planning and knowing how to structure essays, literature reviews, reports and case studies will get you off to a good start. Collecting research, organising your notes and establishing your main points and arguments will help you begin to fill in the details bit by bit. Don't expect anything you write to be perfect first time, you can edit, retune and refine, but the most important thing is to get writing!

Reflective questions

- Can you confidently analyse an essay title?
- Do you know the structural differences between essays, reports and case studies?

Suggested further reading

Tips for good science writing:
Medical Research Council (2021) The secrets of science writing, https://mrc.ukri.org/ skills-careers/studentships/for-current-mrc-students/max-perutz-science-writing- award/the-secrets-of-science-writing/ (accessed 22 June 2021).
If you want to brush up on your grammar skills:
Dignall, C. (2011) *Can You Eat Shoot and Leave? (Workbook).* New York: Collins.
For guidance on literature searching:
Hickson M (2018) *Research Handbook for healthcare professionals.* Oxford: Wiley Black- well.

Reference

Peterson, T.C., Kleppner, S.R. and Botham, C.M. (2018) Ten simple rules for scientists: improving your writing productivity, *PLoS Computational Biology* 14(10): e1006379. https://doi.org/10.1371/journal.pcbi.1006379.

3 Data collection and presentation

Overview and outline

During your degree you will undertake practical sessions where you collect data and subsequently write up a practical report. Likewise, many of you will complete a project for your dissertation that requires data collection. This chapter could require several books in itself; however, our aim is to introduce you to data collection and presentation and increase your confidence to develop your skills in this area.

The skills you will gain by actively collecting data and presenting your findings are exceptionally useful in the real world as there are many scenarios where nutritionists and dietitians do exactly this; see a few selected examples below.

- A supermarket report: '97% of our own-brand products meet Public Health England's salt reduction targets' (Sainsbury's 2021).
- A survey of children's menu options for a Public Health publication: '68% of younger children's fast food and full-service restaurant meals contained more total fat than recommended and more than four times the amount of saturated fat' (Young et al. 2019).
- A clinical audit: '70% of patients had the Malnutrition Universal Screening Tool (MUST) completed correctly. An audit of malnutrition screening across hospital wards.' (Frank et al. 2015).
- Dietetic outcomes report: 'Patients with chronic kidney disease, who met with a renal dietitian twice had a significant improvement in their blood levels of potassium' (Gardiner et al. 2019).

Registered nutritionists and dietitians undertake evidence-based practice, and it is the published research studies that provide the evidence. Understanding study design and data collection is fundamental to understanding the evidence base for the dietary guidelines and knowledge that we have as nutritionists and dietitians. During your degree you will develop the skills needed to find and critically appraise published research studies and decide if and how they can inform your practice (see Chapter 4). Our aim here is to assist you with understanding study design, different types of data and promoting consideration for your intended audience when presenting data.

Introduction to research studies

We will look first at qualitative and quantitative research studies and the different study types you are likely to need to know about.

Qualitative research studies

These tend to investigate how and why individuals act in certain ways and what their views are of various situations. They will involve interviewing participants with analysis-generating themes and presenting quotes (Swift and Tischler 2010). An example of the presentation of qualitative data is shown in the box below.

Themes related to hospital appointments: 37 adults were interviewed and six themes emerged.

Patient concerns	
• Needing to arrange time off work for appointment	• Car parking: finding a space, payment method
• Cancelled/change of date and waiting times	• Cost of parking and travel to appointment
• Lack of privacy; feelings of unease	• Quality of interaction: poor eye contact, excess jargon

(Adapted from Muhammad et al. 2021)

'...think the hospital car park is a serious main issue ... costly and always eager to charge more ... that is the real issue ...with clinical appointments.' Participant 14

Quantitative research studies

These involve collecting data in order to answer a research question. The emphasis is on what is measurable and numerical results are analysed. It is generally not feasible to collect data from an entire population, therefore study investigators collect data on a sample of individuals who are representative of the population. We will highlight some of the main study types that you need to be aware of.

Observational studies including epidemiological studies

These require the study investigators to observe and collect information then report their findings. We highlight a selection of different types of dietary observational studies below.

Cross-sectional studies collect all information from each participant at one time point. This type of study provides a snapshot in time about the population studied.

* Example: 4,738 adults in the UK completed 4-day food diaries as part of the National Diet and Nutrition Survey (NDNS). Tree nut consumers (n=484) had significantly higher intake of vitamin E (11.6 mg) compared with non-consumers (9.8 mg) (Dikariyanto et al. 2020).

Case-control studies require investigators to select a group of individuals who have the outcome of interest (cases). The investigator then selects a second group of individuals (controls), who are similar to the case individuals but do not have the outcome of interest. The investigators look at historical factors to identify if some exposure is found more commonly in the cases than the controls (retrospective data collection).

* Example: people with early onset colorectal cancer (n=175) (the cases) and age-matched controls (n=253) were recruited. Historic information was collected by participants recalling their dietary intake 2 years prior to the study. Greater consumption of sugary drinks ($\geq$ 7 vs. < 1 drinks/week), and a more Westernised dietary pattern were associated with an increased risk of early onset colorectal cancer (Chang et al. 2021).

Prospective longitudinal/cohort studies involve recruitment of healthy participants who are followed up for a period of time and disease and health measurements are reported during the follow up period.

* Example: 22,035 men and women from the general population, where fish consumption was low, were followed for an average of 19 years. During the study period the participants completed dietary intake questionnaires at regular time points. Over the 19 years 1,562 coronary heart disease (CHD) deaths were recorded in the study participants. A protective relationship between fish oil supplement use and CHD deaths was observed (Lentjes et al. 2017).

Intervention or experimental studies – here the investigators intervene to affect the outcome. For example, in a group of 50 participants, 25 would be allocated diet A and the other 25 participants would be allocated diet B, and the same measurements would be taken from the participants. Interventions can be anything from a vitamin supplement to instructions to follow a specific diet or a lifestyle community-based intervention. The study duration can be from a few hours to many months. These studies provide an important evidence base for establishing the link between nutrition and health or illness. See the examples below.

- Example: 630 infants at high risk of peanut allergy were recruited; half were required to avoid peanuts until the age of 3 years, the other half were required to regularly consume peanuts until 3 years of age. At the end of the study 13.7 per cent of the infants avoiding peanuts developed an allergy to peanuts, whereas only 1.9 per cent of the infants regularly consuming peanuts developed a peanut allergy (Du Toit et al. 2015).
- Example: 306 adults with type 2 diabetes were recruited, half the participants (intervention group) were allocated to a very low-calorie weight management programme with food reintroduction and support for weight loss maintenance over a period of 12 months. The other half of participants received usual clinical care (control group). Diabetes remission was achieved in significantly more participants in the intervention group (46 per cent) compared with 4 per cent in the control group (Lean et al. 2017).

Activity

Find the following study and try to answer the questions that follow:
   Muhammad *et al.* (2017) Adherence to a gluten free diet is associated with receiving gluten free foods on prescription and understanding food labelling. *Nutrients,* 97(7): 705. https://doi.org/10.3390/nu9070705
   HINT. The relevant information will be found in the methods section.

- Is it qualitative or quantitative research?
- If it is quantitative, what type of study is it, observational or intervention?
- If it is observational, what type? Cross sectional, case-control or a cohort study?

Reflect. Are you more confident in recognising different study types? You can practise by finding published studies and working out what type of study they are using the information above and exploring the further resources at the end of this chapter.

Data collection

Let's start with: what is data? Data often comprise numeric values from observations/measurements; for example age, energy intake, body weight or quality of life questionnaire scores from participants. These values are termed variables and, for analysis of data, it is useful to categorise the types of data we collect. See Fig. 3.1 for examples of different types of variables. Data is usually inputted into a computer software package and statistical analysis can be undertaken; you will have access to a range of different software through your university course, and you will receive software-specific guidance. Here we

Figure 3.1 Different types of data variables

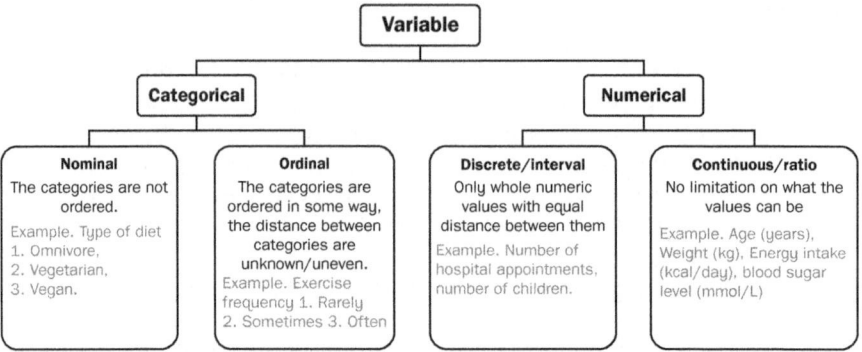

will go over general terms to help build your confidence in understanding what the data is that you have collected.

How you present data depends on the type of data you have collected

Categorical data (nominal and ordinal) is usually presented as the number and percentage of participants from the study population who tick each category. To analyse nominal and ordinal data on a computer, researchers assign numbers to the words (for example, omnivore=1, vegetarian =2, vegan=3), this will enable the software to generate the percentage for each category, and further statistical analysis that may be relevant.

- Example of nominal data presentation. A study of UK adults included 90,742 regular meat-eaters (45.4 per cent), 97,124 low meat-eaters (48.6 per cent), 2,259 poultry-eaters (1.1 per cent), 5,701 fish-eaters (2.9 per cent), 3,870 vegetarians (1.9 per cent), and 248 vegans (0.1 per cent) (Bradbury et al. 2017).
- Example of ordinal data presentation. In response to counting how many portions of fruit and vegetables were eaten from the National Diet and Nutrition Survey (NDNS), only 8 per cent of teenagers met the 5 a day recommendation for fruit and vegetables (Public Health England 2020).

Numerical data (discrete and continuous) is often presented as the average. The most commonly used types of average are the mean and median. The average is presented because it is very difficult to comprehend what all the individual numbers are showing unless it is summarised in a meaningful way. Observed numeric data also have variation; for example, in a sample of 100 adults there will be many different body weight values, and this is termed the variance or spread of the data. The commonly used measurement presenting the spread of data are mean with standard deviation or median with inter-quartile range; we explain these with examples below.

- Sugar-sweetened soft drinks are a major contributor to free sugars intakes. The UK National Diet and Nutrition Survey reported that the highest mean consumption of sugar-sweetened soft drinks was seen in 11- to 18-year-olds (mean ± standard deviation, 142 ± 199 g/day) (Public Health England 2020).
- Gluten-free dietary knowledge score was lower before the telephone intervention (median; interquartile range 13.5; 12.0–14.0) compared with 3 months afterwards (15.0; 14.0–16.0) (Muhammad et al. 2020).

Whether 'mean' or 'median' is used to present your data depends first on whether the data has a normal distribution. If the data is normally distributed, data will usually be presented as mean and standard deviation. Whereas if the data does not follow a normal distribution, it is usually presented as the median and interquartile range. Guidance on how to determine if your data is normally distributed can be found in a statistics textbook, such as those suggested in the further reading list at the end of this chapter.

Variance/spread of the data collected

Examples of presenting numeric data It may have been a while since your last maths lesson, so to assist you in your understanding of averages and variance, we will take you back to the basics with an example using 24-hour energy intake values. The mean is calculated by adding up all the values and dividing this sum by the number of values (e.g. participants). For example, 9 people completed a 24-hour dietary recall and their energy intake was calculated; their data is in table 3.1 below, in participant order.

Table 3.1 Calculation of energy intake following 24-hour dietary recall

Participants	Energy intake Kcal/day
Participant 1	2,850
Participant 2	2,590
Participant 3	2,310
Participant 4	2,160
Participant 5	2,640
Participant 6	2,070
Participant 7	2,320
Participant 8	2,450
Participant 9	2,190

2,850 + 2,590 + 2,310 + 2,160 + 2,640 + 2,070 + 2,320 + 2,450 + 2,190 = 21,580
21,580 divided by 9 (the number of participants) = the study group mean energy intake was 2,398 kcal/day.

A commonly used method of presenting the spread of the numeric values is to determine how much each of the observations are different to the mean value: the standard deviation. The standard deviation is calculated using a specific formula to provide a single value, the larger the value the greater the variation in the values.

The same 9 people completed a 24-hour dietary recall 2 months later.

Task: Look at the individual and mean energy intakes values for the 1st and 2nd 24-hour dietary recalls in table 3.2 below. Can you spot any differences?

Table 3.2   After 9 months: calculation of energy intake following 24-hour dietary recall

Participants	1st energy intake Kcal/day	2nd energy intake Kcal/day
Participant 1	2,850	3,500
Participant 2	2,590	2,100
Participant 3	2,310	2,310
Participant 4	2,160	2,160
Participant 5	2,640	3,000
Participant 6	2,070	1,500
Participant 7	2,320	2,320
Participant 8	2,450	1,600
Participant 9	2,190	2,190
MEAN	**2,398**	**2,398**
Standard deviation	**256**	**588**

Answer. The mean values are the same; however, there are some big changes in the energy intake for 4 individuals. This is summarised by the much larger standard deviation value for the 2nd 24-hour dietary recall compared with the 1st.

Figure 3.2 Illustration to show the mean and the standard deviation

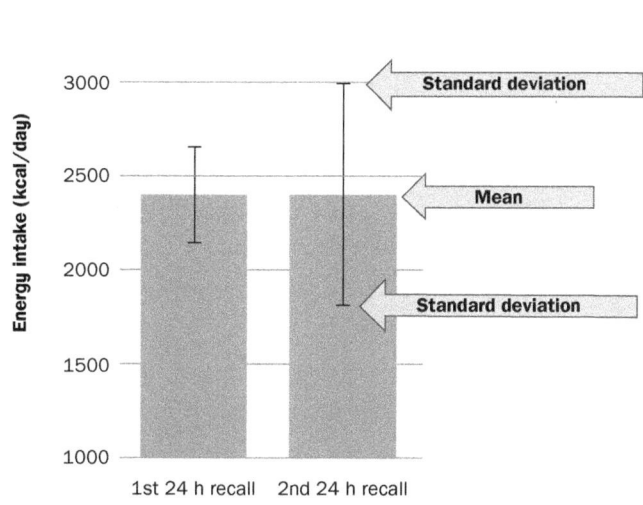

Median and inter quartile range

The median is the middle value if all the values are in order. Now we have our data in order of magnitude in table 3.3, if we consider the middle value, the median, this is also termed the 50th percentile; half the values are lower and half the values are higher (two groups of data). If we split the data into four groups, we have the 25th, 50th and 75th percentile values. The interquartile range is the difference between the 25th and 75th percentile values. Computer software can

Table 3.3 Calculation of energy intake following 24-hour dietary recall, ordered from lowest to highest

Participants	Energy intake Kcal/day
Participant 6	2,070
Participant 4	2,160
Participant 9	2,190
Participant 3	2,310
Participant 7	2,320 ←
Participant 8	2,450
Participant 2	2,590
Participant 5	2,640
Participant 1	2,850

Figure 3.3 Graph to illustrate median and percentiles

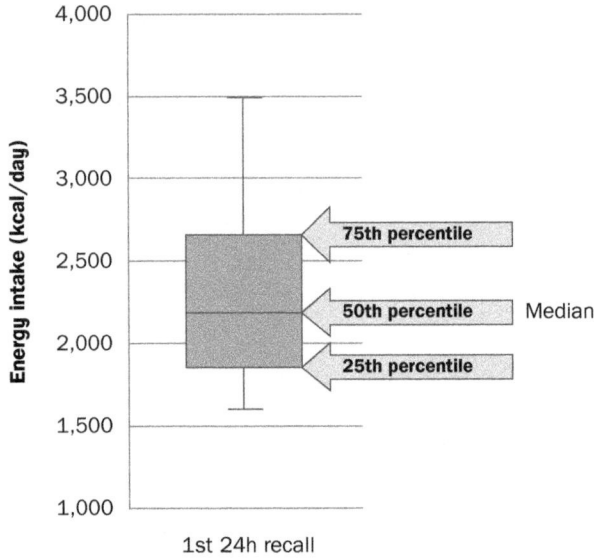

1st 24h recall

calculate the median and interquartile values without you needing to reorder your data; however, we have done this in Table 3.3 to help your understanding of the concept. Using the same study as in the example above, this time the energy intake values are ordered from lowest to highest energy intake.

Now you will be starting to become familiar with the differing study designs and the different types of data that are collected. This is relevant to your student assignments as you will need to be able to understand what type of data you have collected and how you will present it and what, if any statistical analysis to undertake.

Activity

Continuing with the Muhammad et al. (2017) study from the task earlier in this chapter, see if you can find out how they present their findings. Do they use mean and standard deviation or median with interquartile ranges?

Muhammad et al. (2017) Adherence to a gluten free diet is associated with receiving gluten free foods on prescription and understanding food labelling. *Nutrients*, 97(7): 705. https://doi.org/10.3390/nu9070705

HINT. The relevant information will be found in the results section.

Introduction to choosing a statistical test

As students, and as Associate Registered Nutritionists and Dietitians, you will want to know if there is a relationship between two variables or if there is a

Table 3.4 Commonly used statistical tests

Data type	Statistical test(s)	Example
Categorical data	Chi squared test	Are there more male vegans than female vegans? *Data needed: number of vegans and number of males and females in the study. Number of male and female vegans and non vegans in the study.*
Two groups with numeric data	Independent t-test Mann Whitney U Test	Do young children eat more portions of vegetables per day than adolescents? *Data needed: a group of young children and a group of adolescents, all need to provide information on how many portions of vegetables they consume per day.*
Numeric values from participants at two time points	Paired t-test Wilcoxon signed ranks test	Do participants lose weight after an intervention? *Data needed: weights of participants before and after the intervention.*
Two sets of numeric data	Pearson's correlation Spearman's correlation	Is there a relationship with dietary fish oil intake and breast milk fatty acid composition? *Data needed: fish oil intake data and samples of breast milk analysed for fatty acids.*
		Is there a relationship between dietary knowledge and behaviour? *Data needed: dietary knowledge score and a behaviour score.*

difference in outcome between two different dietary treatments. Statistical tests are a tool to establish if the relationship, or difference that you think is there, is the result of chance or if there is a strong possibility that it is a real difference or relationship (summary of common statistical test in Table 3.4). In other words, is the information you have collected from your study sample able to be generalised to the wider population Statistics are all about probability: what is the likelihood of the same result occurring again in the same/similar circumstances? Statistical tests provide a selection of important values, one of them being the p value. If a difference/or relationship is highly probable the p value will be reported as less than 0.05 (<0.05).

We have provided you with the briefest of introductions to statistical tests. This is a starting point so you can start to appreciate their place in data collection and presentation. Their inclusion is to assist in enabling you to move onto greater understanding within your degree and to utilise the further reading outlined at the end of the chapter.

Presenting data: text, tables and graphs

Clear presentation of your data is key to demonstrating your understanding of the data you have collected as part of a university assignment. As an Associate Registered Nutritionist or Dietitian, clearly presenting data is a major part of being able to communicate information to your chosen audience. This could be the public, other healthcare professionals or people paying for a service.

The visual presentation of data is a powerful tool for conveying information about the data you have collected. Developing your confidence and skills in presenting data for university reports, presentations and in your career is obviously important. The text, tables and graphs should be complementary, each contributing to the overall message to the reader/audience reading your report. It is rarely necessary to repeat information within tables and graphs; the graphs should be used to highlight key findings from the data.

- Example. The information presented below is from the same cross-sectional study, and is presented within a paragraph of text, a table (Table 3.5) and a graph (Fig. 3.4). What do you notice when looking at the same information presented in different ways?

'Forty-four lean women with polycystic ovary syndrome (PCOS) and 38 healthy lean women (controls) completed a questionnaire on eating behaviour. The average binge eating symptom scores from lean women with PCOS (mean ± standard deviation: 10.9 ± 7.8) was significantly higher compared with the average score from healthy controls (7.4 ± 6.0, p<0.01).' (Jeanes et al. 2017).

Table 3.5   Binge eating scores from lean women with and without polycystic ovary syndrome (PCOS)

	Healthy n=38	PCOS n=44
Binge eating symptom score* Mean ± standard deviation	**7.4 ± 6.0**	**10.9 ± 7.8**[a]
Absence of both compulsive eating and binge-eating.	65% n=26	50% n=22
Unusual eating pattern might be a compulsive eater who eats excessively but does not binge-eat.	17.5% n=7	13.6% n=6
Subclinical group of binge-eaters, either in the initial stages of the disorder or recovered bulimics.	5.0% n=2	15.9% n=7
Highly disordered eating pattern and the presence of binge-eating.	7.5% n=3	20.5% n=9

[a] Significant difference between healthy and PCOS women (p<0.01); independent t-test.
* Possible range for binge-eating symptom score (0–30). (Jeanes et al. 2017).

Figure 3.4 Binge-eating scores from lean women with and without polycystic ovary syndrome (PCOS). Data presented as mean with standard deviations, significant difference in scores; p<0.01 (Jeanes et al. 2017)

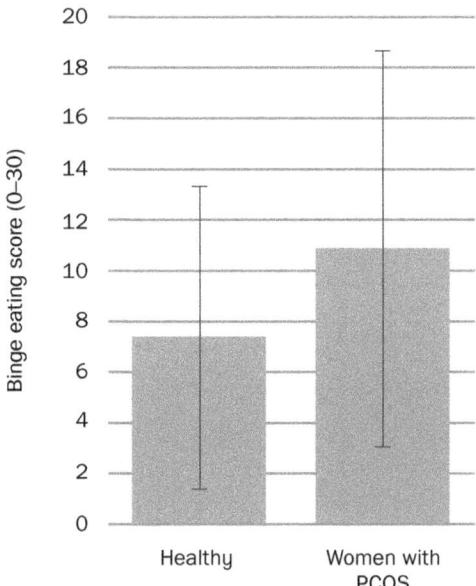

You will notice from the example above that it is a lot quicker and easier to see the difference in binge eating scores from the figure (and the large variance/ spread of the values), compared to reading the text; however, there is a lot more useful information presented within the table.

The role of text is to lead the reader through the important findings; tables can present a lot of information together and the figure emphasises the important data to the reader.

The following tips can improve the quality of your report/findings:
- Use clearly presented tables and/or figures to break up the text and emphasise key information.
- Make sure your tables and figures are labelled with a useful description.
- Include the units within your figure and table.
- If you have done a statistical test, include the p value(s) within your table or figure.
- Check that you have referred to your table(s) and figure(s) within your text.

Tables are a very useful way of presenting a lot of numeric data in a small amount of space or restricted word allowance. A well-presented table can enable the reader to quickly and clearly see many results, and you can demonstrate your ability to select and present data appropriately. The information within a table does not need to be repeated in text; however, it is important to pick out one or two key points and refer to the table.

- Example 1. 'Beverages contributed between a quarter and a third of all sugars consumed, with boys aged 9–10 years consuming the most sugar in total' (Coppinger et al. 2013) shown in Table 3.6.

Table 3.6 Mean daily total sugar and sugar from beverages intake

Age and gender	Total sugar (g/day)	Sugar from beverages (g/day)
9–10 years, boys (n=29)	155 ± 61	35 ± 14
11–13 years, boys (n=95)	110 ± 76	35 ± 59
9–10 years, girls (n=41)	129 ± 67	33 ± 19
11–13 years, girls (n=85)	101 ± 58	27 ± 20

(Based on data from Coppinger et al. 2013)

- Example 2. 'Serum 25 (OH) vitamin D values at 24 months were significantly greater compared with values prior to surgery' (Table 3.8) (Gillon et al. 2017).

Table 3.7 Blood micronutrient values prior to and 24 months post-bariatric surgery

	n	Pre-operative	24 months post-operative	P value
25 (OH) vitamin D (mmol/L)	164	47 ± 28	59 ± 21 0	0.002
Ferritin (īg/L)	229	116 ± 107	88 ± 96	<0.001
Folate (nmol/L)	228	14.3 ± 8.0	18.2 ± 11.0	<0.001
Vitamin B12 (pmol/L)	234	318 ± 144	326 ± 224	0.566

(Based on data from Gillon et al. 2017)

Within your practical class or dissertation, you may collect a lot of data, and working out the best ways to present it within a table can take quite a bit of time. Look at published studies and see how they have presented data that is similar to the data you have collected; this is a good way to develop your awareness of the many different ways of presenting results within a table.

A graph (figure) provides the reader with a visual impression of the content and meaning of your results. Graphs come in many different forms, and with computer software you have numerous options available to you. A well thought out and presented graph will demonstrate understanding of your data, and combine simplicity, accuracy and clarity.

General rules
- Categorical data: pie chart or bar chart
- Numeric data from different groups: bar chart
- Numeric data over time: line graph

Figure 3.5 Proportion of students in different weight categories as a pie chart and a bar graph

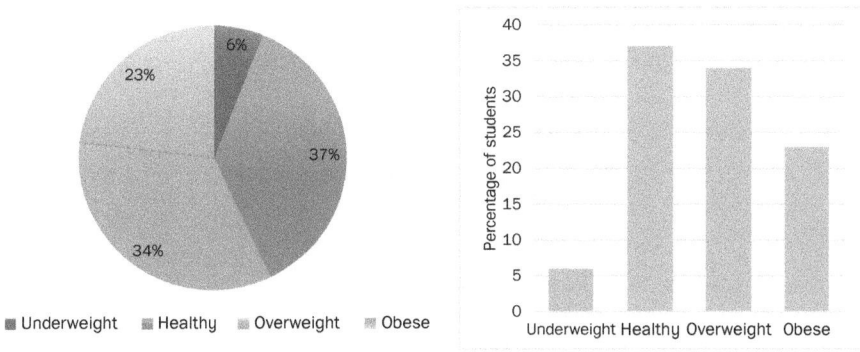

Both the pie chart and the bar graph (Fig. 3.5) clearly illustrate the small proportion of participants who were underweight (BMI <18.5 kgm^{-2}) and the much larger proportion who were overweight or obese. From this, you can begin to appreciate that sometimes there is not a right or wrong answer; it is your personal opinion on which you choose to include.

Top tip: Give yourself enough time to organise your data and present it well. If you are not familiar with making graphs it can take longer than you expect.

Consider the axis that would be optimal for your data. In the example below (Fig. 3.6) the results look dramatically different. A dietary intervention to reduce the glycaemic index of the diet was undertaken and the glycaemic index of the diet was calculated from 3-day food diaries at week 0 and week 12. Figure 3.6A is showing a substantial difference whereas Fig. 3.6B appears to show little difference. Look a little closer at the y axis and you may be able to spot that in fact the same data is presented, just using a different scale on the y axis. There was in fact a significant reduction in glycaemic index values (data adapted from Barr et al. 2013).

Scatter plot graphs provide a visual of a potential relationship between two continuous variables. In the example below you can clearly see the relationship between salt intake and blood pressure in Fig. 3.7B, whereas in Fig. 3.7A, it is a lot more difficult.

Figure 3.6   Glycaemic index of the diet at base line and week 12, using different scales (data from Barr et al. 2013)

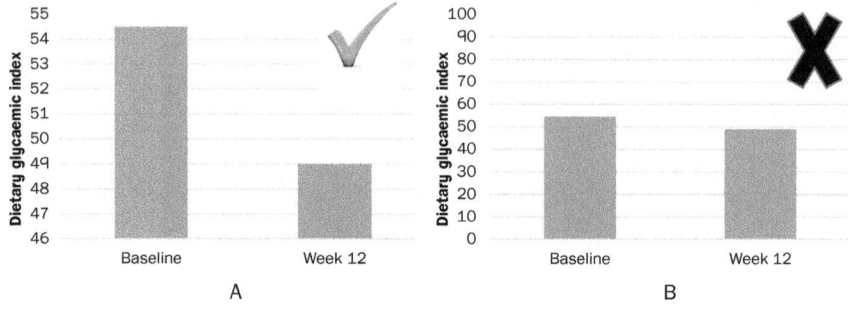

Figure 3.7   Scatter plots showing the relationship between salt intake and blood pressure

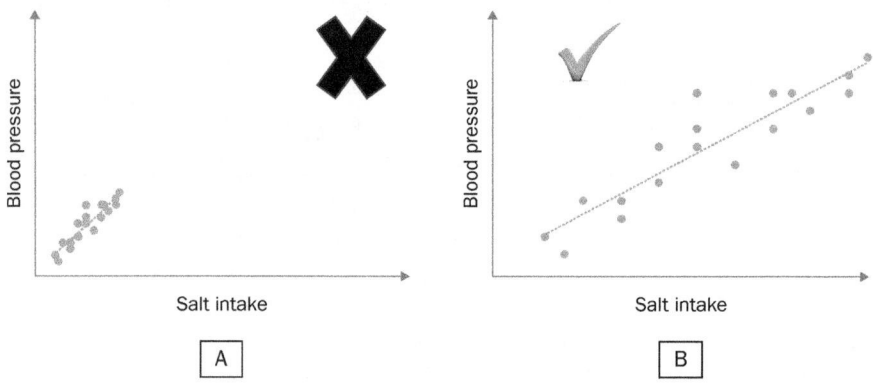

It may take several attempts to change your axes, ensure they are labelled and get your graphs optimal but, if it displays your data clearly, it will be worth the effort.

Summary

Within this chapter we have introduced you to study design, different types of data (categorical and numerical) and touched on some basic statistical terms. Understanding study design and the types of data collected are fundamental skills to interpret the results from published studies and ultimately design your own audit, service evaluation or research project.

You will have the opportunity, within your degree, to collect and present data. We have given you guidance and ideas for how to present the data you collect as part of a university practical or dissertation. This is valuable experience as with your career as a registered nutritionist or dietitian there will be many times when these skills are required.

Reflective questions

- Can you explain the difference between qualitative and quantitative studies?
- Do you know how the mean and median values differ?
- Are you aware of the benefits of different ways to present data?

Suggested further reading

Hickson, M. (2018) *Research Handbook for Healthcare Professionals*. Oxford: Wiley Blackwell.

Lovegrove, J.A., Hodson, L., Sharma, S. and Lanham-New, S.A. (2015) *Nutrition Research Methodologies*. Nutrition Society Textbook. Oxford: Wiley Blackwell.

Petrie, A. and Sabin, C. (2019) *Medical Statistics at a Glance*, 4th edn. Oxford: Wiley Blackwell.

Willet, W. (2012) *Nutritional Epidemiology*, 3rd edn. Oxford: Oxford University Press.

References

Barr, S., Reeves, S., Sharp, K. and Jeanes, Y. (2013) An isocaloric low glycaemic diet improves metabolic profile in women with polycystic ovary syndrome, *Journal of the Academy of Nutrition and Dietetics*, 113: 1523–31.

Bradbury, K.E., Tong, T. and Key, T. (2017) Dietary intake of high-protein foods and other major foods in meat-eaters, poultry-eaters, fish-eaters, vegetarians, and vegans in UK Biobank, *Nutrients*, 9(12): 1317. https://doi.org/10.3390/nu9121317

Chang, V.C., Cotterchio, M., De, P. and Tinmouth, J. (2021) Risk factors for early-onset colorectal cancer: a population-based case-control study in Ontario, Canada, *Cancer Causes Control*, doi: 10.1007/s10552-021-01456-8. Epub ahead of print. PMID: 34120288.

Coppinger, T., Jeanes, Y., Mitchell, M. and Reeves, S. (2013) Beverage consumption and BMI of British schoolchildren aged 9–13 years, *Public Health Nutrition* 16: 1244–49.

Dikariyanto, V., Berry, S., Pot, G. et al. (2020) Tree nut snack consumption is associated with better diet quality and CVD risk in the UK adult population: National Diet and Nutrition Survey 2008–2014, *Public Health Nutrition*: 23: 3160–69.

Du Toit, G., Roberts, G., Sayre, P.H. et al. (2015) Randomized trial of peanut consumption in infants at risk for peanut allergy, *New England Journal of Medicine*, 372: 803–13.

Frank, M., Sivagnanaratnam, A. and Bernstein, J. (2015) Nutritional assessment in elderly care: a MUST! *BMJ Open Quality*, 4: u204810.w2031. doi: 10.1136/bmjquality.u204810.w2031

Gardiner, C., El-Sherbini, N., Perry, S. et al. (2019) The Renal Dietetic Outcome Tool (RDOT) in clinical practice, *Journal of Kidney Care*, 4: 116–24.

Gillon, S., Jeanes, Y., Andersen, J.R. and Villy, V. (2017) Micronutrient status in morbidly obese patients prior to laparoscopic sleeve gastrectomy and micronutrient changes 5 years' post-surgery, *Obesity Surgery*, 27: 606–12.

Jeanes, Y., Reeves, S., Gibson, E.I. et al. (2017) Binge eating behaviours and food cravings in women with Polycystic Ovary Syndrome, *Appetite*, 109: 29–32.

Lean, M.E.J., Leslie, W.S., Barnes, A.C. et al. (2017) Primary care-led weight management for remission of type 2 diabetes (DiRECT): an open-label cluster-randomised trial, *The Lancet*, https://doi.org/10.1016/S0140-6736(17)33102-1.

Lentjes, M.A.H., Keogh, R.H., Welch, A.A. et al. (2017) Longitudinal associations between marine omega-3 supplement users and coronary heart disease in a UK population-based cohort. *BMJ Open*, 7(10): e017471. doi: 10.1136/bmjopen-2017-017471

Muhammad, H., Reeves, S., Ishaq, S. et al. (2020) Telephone clinic improves gluten-free dietary adherence in adults with coeliac disease: sustained at 6 months. *Frontline Gastroenterology*, October 2020. doi:10.1136/flgastro-2020-101643

Muhammad, H., Reeves, S., Ishaq, S. and Jeanes Y. (2021) Experiences of outpatient clinics and opinions of telehealth by Caucasian and South Asian patients with celiac disease. *Journal of Patient Experience*, January 2021. doi:10.1177/23743735211018083

Public Health England (2020) National Diet and Nutrition Survey. Available at: https://assets.publishing.service.gov.uk/government/uploads/system/uploads/attachment_data/file/943114/NDNS_UK_Y9-11_report.pdf (accessed 9 November 2021).

Sainsbury's (2021) Health. Available at: https://about.sainsburys.co.uk/making-a-difference/netzero/diets/health (accessed 02 July 2021).

Swift, J.A. and Tischler, V. (2010) Qualitative research in nutrition and dietetics: getting started, *Journal of Human Nutrition and Dietetics*, 23(6): 559–66. doi: http://dx.doi.org/10.1111/j.1365-277X.2010.01116.x

Young, M., Coppinger, T. and Reeves, S. (2019). The nutritional value of children's meals in chain restaurants in the UK and Ireland, *Journal of Nutrition Education and Behaviour*, 51, 817–25.

4 Evidence and referencing

Overview and outline

There are many different sources of information that you will come across during your degree; while some may be from peer-reviewed journals, other sources may even be on social media. Regardless, you need to be able to judge the source of that information and be able to make scientific judgements based on the quality and accuracy of the information you are presented with. You will also need to ensure you reference any material you refer to appropriately and avoid the risk of plagiarism. This chapter will outline how to identify reliable sources of information, read and critique journal articles, paraphrase and summarise in your own words and then reference materials in the correct manner.

Introduction

A key skill for a Dietitian or an Associate Registered Nutritionist is to be able to source information and assess its suitability. For example, whilst an article you came across in a magazine might be an interesting read, you would not quote it in an essay or give a patient advice from it. Therefore, it is extremely important that you can judge the quality of information and assess its accuracy and reliability, before moving on to evaluate it and critique it.

How to read a research paper

Engaging with the scientific literature and keeping up to date on new publications is essential and journal papers can provide knowledge but also opportunities for critique. It is important to read and evaluate research papers, as you will use these skills a lot when writing essays and reports. The Quality Assurance Agency for UK degrees (QAA 2019) considers these important graduate skills and have described them in their benchmark standards as shown in Table 4.1.

Table 4.1 QAA Benchmark standards for sourcing and appraising the academic literature

Level	Threshold	Typical	Excellent
Description	Be able to source academic literature and extract relevant points.	Critically appraise academic literature and other sources of information.	Demonstrate a highly developed ability for critical appraisal of academic literature and other sources of information.

(QAA 2021)

Whilst clearly important, we recognise that journal papers are not always the easiest things to read, and in the words of Ruben (2016): *'Nothing makes you feel stupid quite like reading a scientific journal article'*.

However, there are a few things you can do to change that feeling:

- **Scan the paper, read it and then re-read it** – re-read it as many times as you like.
- **You may want to prioritise certain sections of the paper** – research by Hubbard and Dunbar (2017) found that sometimes inexperienced readers found the methods and results sections the most challenging to read, and you may want to read those particular sections several times over.
- **Look at the figures** – don't skim over the tables and graphs, often these are key to the whole paper so take time to check the details about what they are showing.
- **Identify key ideas in the paper** – how would you summarise this paper if describing it to a friend, what was the main finding that the authors reported?
- **Read critically** – have the results been put in context and what are the limitations of the findings? The authors themselves may have also included a section in the paper on the limitations of their research, usually towards the end of the discussion paragraph.
- **Give it time to let it sink in** – sometimes coming back to a paper the next day can give you a fresh perspective.
- **Sometimes papers are just badly written!** – so don't be too hard on yourself if you are struggling to understand a particular paper. But do think about what you could do to fully understand it. Sometimes just writing a list of the commonly used acronyms can help, or perhaps you need to look up what certain terms or concepts mean before you can continue with that particular paper. Perhaps you could ask someone else to go through it with you and get their perspective on it.
- **Keep practising** – as with all things, the more you do it the better you will get at it.

> **Challenge**
> Could you read one scientific journal paper a day for a whole month?

Evaluating information

Being able to judge the quality and reliability of information is key and one way of assessing the source of any information is to apply what is known as the 'CRAAP test' (Meriam Library 2010). This test is based on five questions that you can ask yourself when trying to decide if an information source is credible and reliable. The five questions are shown in Table 4.2.

Table 4.2 The CRAAP test explained

Key questions	Supplementary questions
Is it **C**urrent?	Has this information been published recently?
Is it **R**eliable?	Where was the article or information published; was it a peer-reviewed journal or was it on a blog?
Who was the **A**uthor?	Was it written by an individual or an organisation or even a marketing company?
Is it **A**ccurate?	Has the article been reviewed and is there any evidence or data for the claims that are made?
What was its **P**urpose?	Why was it written and published and who is it aimed at?

Source: based on information from the Meriam Library (2010).

Peer-reviewed journals

Good sources of information with relevance to the study and practice of nutrition and dietetics are going to be peer-reviewed journals. Peer review means that the papers have been submitted to a journal and then scrutinised by experts from the same subject area. This helps ensure that unsubstantiated claims or personal biases are not presented and that data collection and experiments have been conducted scientifically and ethically. This also means that peer-reviewed articles can generally be considered a more trusted form of scientific communication (Kelly et al. 2014).

Identifying fake news

In the fields of nutrition and dietetics there is plenty of anecdotal information that we need to be aware of. But what works for one person does not necessarily mean it should be recommended to others; indeed it might not even be true. One research study found that when it comes to anecdotes and social media, false news spreads faster and further than genuine news (Riis et al. 2019). Be wary of online information: some sites are more reputable than others, and this includes Wikipedia. Doubtless you will have come across this online encyclopaedia, but did you know it can be edited by anyone? In many cases it is compiled by people who are specialists in their field, but this also means it could be written by someone who may not have the most accurate nor up-to-date information; so be very cautious. Therefore, it is important that you are able to spot any fake news. You can avoid misinformation by using the CRAAP test as described above, but other points you may want to consider include the following (Central Michigan Libraries 2021):

- Checking the source of that information.
- Don't just read the headlines – they could be click bait.
- Checking your biases: often we want to believe something is true.
- Check the author (are they real?) and the date (is it an old news story?).
- Is it a joke?
- If in any doubt, ask an expert.

Hierarchy of evidence

Both Dietitians and Registered Nutritionists are required to ensure their practice is evidence based but, in order to do this, it is essential to have access to and recognise high-quality information. Information quality can be categorised in many ways. One method of sorting different sources of information is according to the hierarchy of evidence (an example of a pyramid that depicts the hierarchy of evidence can be seen in Fig. 4.1). This information has been presented in many different ways and there are many different versions of

Figure 4.1 Hierarchy of evidence pyramid

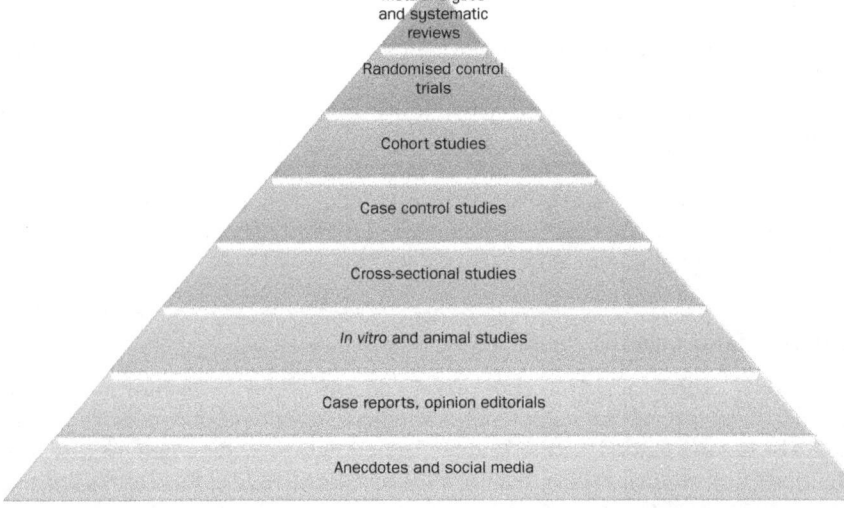

Meta-analyses and systematic reviews

Randomised control trials

Cohort studies

Case control studies

Cross-sectional studies

In vitro and animal studies

Case reports, opinion editorials

Anecdotes and social media

these pyramids (e.g. Howick et al. 2011; Murad et al. 2016; Tomlin and Borgetto 2011). Essentially, it means organising evidence from the weakest to strongest. At the base of the pyramid is the flimsiest forms of evidence, such as something you might read on social media or an anecdote, whereas at the top of the pyramid are the meta-analyses; these are papers where data from multiple studies have been combined and analysed statistically. Because they are based on several studies they are said to have improved statistical power compared to the original individual studies (Ismail 2016). In between you have the cohort studies, case control studies, cross-sectional studies, *in vitro* and animal studies, followed by case reports and opinion-based editorials.

When looking at the hierarchy of evidence pyramid there are a few other points to consider.

- Even the strongest forms of evidence can be performed poorly.
- There is still a need for some of the weaker forms of evidence, for example cross-sectional studies; not least as starting points for more powerful designs; you need several studies to be able to conduct a meta-analysis and many studies to be able to conduct a systematic review.

Critiquing what you have read

Critical thinking is a key skill that you will develop during your time at university. Just as you will need to be able to assess good sources of information, you must also ask questions with an open mind about what you have read so you can assess different arguments for and against particular points. You can then use the evidence provided to back up your views and theories. This will include ensuring you have the facts correct, using logical reasoning to deduce answers, and perhaps even some awareness of your own biases. It does not mean you should criticise different viewpoints but rather learn to question and evaluate the information and the sources of that information as you develop your own evidence-based ideas, so you can take part in scientific debate. When you are critiquing a study, you are not describing it, you are considering the strengths and weaknesses. Critique does not have to be negative, you can also include positive comments, but given that it is extremely difficult to conduct the perfect piece of research there is usually something in the study that can be critiqued.

Journal clubs

If your university has a journal club, consider joining in. If not, perhaps you could start one yourself? There are also lots of online journal clubs for students. These journal clubs can help you develop your critiquing skills in a friendly and supportive environment.

Referencing

Referencing is the way to acknowledge the sources of information that you use in your assignments. Every time you refer to any information, you must have an in-text citation and a reference in the list at the end acknowledging the author of that information.

Quoting, paraphrasing and summarising

Do you know the difference between quoting, paraphrasing and summarising?

Quoting: It is best to use direct quotes only on rare occasions for something quite unique or exceptional, for example:

'There is no love sincerer than the love of food' (Shaw 1903).

Then you should include full details about the source of the quote in the reference list at the end:

Shaw, B. (1903) *Man and Superman*. Cambridge, Mass.: The University Press.

However, in most cases it is better if you can to put the information in your own words by either paraphrasing or summarising.

Paraphrasing: is where you put the information into your own words. However, you must still acknowledge the source of the information that you used to inform your words. Paraphrasing is preferred to quoting because it can show you have absorbed and understood the information and then written it in a way that is suited to your writing style. However, this does not mean using a thesaurus to change words so it looks like you have written it, in fact, doing this can change the meaning of the sentence; so take your time to think about what point you want to make and use your own words to do so.

Summarising: usually provides a broader view of the information and can include your own ideas, but you must still acknowledge the original source of the ideas. If you can combine different sources of information even better; it is perfectly fine to use more than one reference for a single point.

When to use et al.

When citing authors in the text it is usual to give the author's surname and the year the work was published, so: (Smith 2022). If there are two authors, it should be like this: (Smith and Jones 2022). However, when there are more than two authors it is common to use et al. *Et al* is short for *et alia*, which is Latin for 'and others'. This means giving the first author's surname and then et al. to show there are more than two authors, for example: (Smith et al. 2022). The full list of authors can be given in the reference list at the end.

Different referencing styles

There are many different referencing styles such as Chicago, Vancouver and American Psychological Association (APA); you may have seen a variety used by different journals and books. However, the one that is most commonly used by university nutrition and dietetic departments, and explained in detail here, is the Harvard style of referencing.

Harvard referencing

Harvard is probably one of the most popular styles of referencing and is often used in journals. Although this is the style most commonly used in universities, some institutions may prefer a slightly modified version of this (for more on this see below and do check with your university).

For in-text citations the author and date is used. So to cite this book you could add (Reeves and Jeanes 2022) in the text after the information you have used. Alternatively, if you want to mention the authors by name as part of your sentence, you could write something like this:

'According to Reeves and Jeanes (2022) …'

Note, in this case only the year is put in brackets.

Remember that any references you cite in the text should be included in the list at the end and you must also check that any references in the list at the end are cited in the text!

Step-by-step guide: listing references for a journal article (Harvard style)

This is how references should be presented in the list at the end of your work.

Give all the authors' names, surname first followed by initials:
Brown, A. and Chen, D.
Then add the year it was written/published:
Brown, A. and Chen, D. (2022)
Include the article title:
Brown, A. and Chen, D. (2022) Sustainable diets around the globe
The journal title is usually in italics:
Brown, A. and Chen, D. (2022) Sustainable diets around the globe, *Clinical Dietetics*
Then add the volume number:
Brown, A. and Chen, D. (2022) Sustainable diets around the globe, *Clinical Dietetics*, 44
Lastly add the page numbers and finish with a full stop
Brown, A. and Chen, D. (2022) Sustainable diets around the globe, *Clinical Dietetics*, 44: 3–12.
If the journal article has been published online only you will need to include the DOI number, as shown below:
Brown, A. and Chen, D. (2022) Sustainable diets around the globe, *Clinical Dietetics* Published online first 06 January 2022 doi: 10.1136/clindiet-2022-101852

Your university may have a slight variation on the Harvard style of referencing so always consult your study guides or check with the library staff. For example, some university styles advocate using a full stop after the year, or include the issue number after the volume number, or pp before the page numbers, as shown here:

Brown, A. and Chen, D. (2022). Sustainable diets around the globe, *Clinical Dietetics*, 44 (3), pp.3–12.

However, for the most part your lecturers will be looking to ensure you have included all the key information and that you are consistent.

Listing references for a book

The above guide was for a journal article, if you want to reference a book you will also need to know:

- The place where the book was published and the name of publisher

For example:

Edris, F. (2022) *Weight Bias in Society*. London: McGraw Hill.

For a chapter in an edited book

Here you will need the author of the chapter and also the name of the book editor. For example:

Giannis, H. (2022) Anthropometry in dietary assessment, in Irwin, J. (ed.) *Current Nutritional Assessment*. Maidenhead: Open University Press, pp. 25–34.

Referencing websites

As with the other references start with the author. If there is no author, then use the corporate name of whoever owns the website content. Do write out the full names rather than the acronyms, e.g. World Health Organization rather than WHO. You should also add the day you accessed the information, as websites are constantly being updated. For example:

Public Health England (2020) *National Diet and Nutrition Survey*. Available at: https://www.gov.uk/government/collections/national-diet-and-nutrition-survey (accessed 26 May 2021).

Remember:

- Your reference list should be listed in alphabetical order according to the first author's surname. For Harvard style you should not use bullet points or numbers.
- Try to reference as you go along; if you leave it to the end, you are more likely to leave references out and make mistakes.
- Be as consistent as possible in your style.
- You are more likely to be marked down for not using enough references than you are for using too many references.

Bibliographies

Bibliographies are slightly different from reference lists in that they include all the information you may have used to complete the assignment including that used for background reading or information purposes; this might include sources that you did not use in the end so therefore did not need to cite in the text. Sometimes you may be required to include a reference list **and** a bibliography but, for most universities, assignments in the field of nutrition and dietetics you will only need a reference list.

Reference management systems

Most universities will have a subscription to some sort of reference management software such as Endnote, Mendeley, Refworks etc. These can be useful to help you save references as you go along, identify those that you want to read or access later, organise your references by topic, insert citations into your essays and papers, and create reference lists in the appropriate style at the end of your essay or paper. They can save you a lot of time and effort.

Avoiding plagiarism

With careful and diligent referencing, it should be possible to avoid accidental plagiarism. However, it is worth making sure you fully understand what plagiarism is so you can ensure you prevent it happening. Plagiarism means academic cheating. Essentially it is an attempt to pass off someone else's work as your own, whether that is intentional or unintentional (Carroll 2007).

There are various levels of plagiarism: it could be a nicely worded phrase, copied and pasted from an online journal paper, or it could be entire essay bought from an essay mill. Whilst the latter is clearly much more serious than the former, all types of plagiarism will be treated seriously and must be avoided.

Penalties for plagiarism depend on the university, the extent of the plagiarism and sometimes the university may give consideration as to whether it is a first or subsequent offence. This might earn you a warning, a fail for that piece of work or, if really serious, it could even result in you being asked to leave the university; therefore it is extremely important that you understand what plagiarism is to avoid ever being in such a situation.

Whilst we recognise that plagiarism is not always deliberate, even accidental plagiarism can be avoided with good study skills

Common errors

These can include the following:

- Using someone else's words
- Putting information in your own words but not giving a reference
- Providing a direct 'quote' but not giving a reference
- Cut and pasting

- Recycling from other pieces of coursework
- Colluding with other students (working together when it is expected that you will write separate reports).

To avoid these errors, you may need to rethink the way you collect information and write your assignments:

- Do you copy and paste chunks from online sources and then try to put that in your words?
- Do you use the thesaurus to change words?
- Do you move sentences around to try and make your writing look different to the original?
- Do you forget to keep a record of references used?

If so, this style of working is likely to be a problem. Instead:

- Always write everything in your own words, even when compiling information and your own notes for your work.
- Think about what points you are trying to make then, without looking at the original source, write those points down. Even though you have written this yourself you must reference the sources from where you got the ideas.
- Don't worry about changing frequently used words or switching words to try to make your writing look different from the original work; this can inadvertently change the meaning of your sentence. There are some words such as 'metabolism' that simply cannot be substituted no matter how many alternative suggestions your thesaurus provides.
- Make sure you cite and list your references as you go along, it will be much easier than trying to do it all at the end and you will be less likely to leave out an essential reference.

These tips will not only ensure you avoid plagiarism but will also ensure your essay/report is written entirely in your own style, that the style is consistent throughout and generally flows well.

Self-plagiarism

Self-plagiarism is where you try to reuse work that you have already submitted. For the most part, in modules where you have a choice of what to write about, you will be advised to choose a topic that you have not written about before. However, there are certain themes such as 'obesity' that will come up in a variety of modules. In such cases, not only should you never submit the same essay for different modules, remember that you should not recycle any part of that essay, since self-plagiarism is usually treated in the same way as other types of plagiarism. This becomes even more important if you get the opportunity to publish your work in a journal, for example, as although technically you may own the intellectual property, the journal is likely to own the publication copyright.

Plagiarism detection software

Most universities use anti-plagiarism software such as 'Turnitin'; such programs allow you to submit your work electronically for marking. But, in addition to being a place for lecturers to provide feedback, the program also compares your work to published sources as well as the work of other students. It is always worth submitting your work early and then looking at the similarity report. If you are allowed resubmissions, you may be able to correct any similarities you may have accidentally made. Do not be put off by a high overall similarity score (although it can indicate a problem), if you have used a lot of references this can increase the overall percentage. For this reason you must look at the actual document to see if there are any similarities there; these will usually be highlighted in a different colour. Whilst these software packages can indicate where you have made mistakes, ideally you will have done all you can to avoid plagiarism in the first place. Take care with your note writing and referencing; but remember that originality and critique will always be the best way to avoid plagiarism.

Summary

As Dietitians and Associate Registered Nutritionists, it is important that you are able to identify suitable sources of evidence-based information and have an insight to the different levels of evidence that exist, when you are evaluating papers. The more you read journal papers and get used to that style of writing, the easier you will find them to understand, so keep reading and critiquing papers. Also it is important to keep a track of any references you use as you go along to avoid the risk of plagiarism in your original work.

Reflective questions

- Can you assess the quality of different information sources?
- Have you checked what style of referencing your university prefers?
- Do you know what plagiarism is and how to avoid it?

Suggested further reading

Hubbard, K.E. and Dunbar, S.D. (2017) Perceptions of scientific research literature and strategies for reading papers depend on academic career stage, *PLoS ONE*, 12(12): e0189753. https://doi.org/10.1371/journal.pone.0189753

Wrigley, S. (2016) How universities can help students avoid plagiarism: get them to write better. *The Conversation*. Available at: https://theconversation.com/how-universities-can-help-students-avoid-plagiarism-get-them-to-write-better-51434 (accessed 2 November 2021).

References

Carroll, J. (2007) *A Handbook for Deterring Plagiarism in Higher Education*, 2nd edn. Oxford: Oxford Centre for Staff Learning and Development.

Central Michigan Libraries (2021) Website research: fake news. Available at: https://libguides.cmich.edu/web_research/fakenews (accessed 26 May 2021).

Howick, J., Chalmers, I., Glasziou, P. et al. (2011). *The 2011 Oxford CEBM Levels of Evidence (Introductory Document)*. Oxford: Oxford Centre for Evidence-Based Medicine. Available at: https://www.cebm.ox.ac.uk/resources/levels-of-evidence/ocebm-levels-of-evidence (accessed 8 June 2021).

Hubbard, K.E. and Dunbar, S.D. (2017) Perceptions of scientific research literature and strategies for reading papers depend on academic career stage, *PLoS ONE*, 12(12): e0189753. https://doi.org/10.1371/journal.pone.0189753.

Ismail, A. (2016) *Meta-analysis: What, Why, and How*. Available at: https://s4be.cochrane.org/blog/2016/12/02/meta-analysis-what-why-and-how/ (accessed 8 June 2021).

Kelly, J., Sadeghieh, T. and Adel, K. (2014) Peer review in scientific publications: benefits, critiques, and a survival guide, *EJIFCC*, 25(3): 227–43.

Meriam Library, California State University-Chico (2010) Evaluating information – applying the CRAAP test. Available at: https://library.csuchico.edu/sites/default/files/craap-test.pdf) (accessed 26 May 2021).

Murad, M.H., Asi, N., Alsawas, M. et al. (2016) New evidence pyramid, *BMJ Evidence-Based Medicine*, 21: 125–27.

Quality Assurance Agency (2021) *Subject Benchmark Statement Agriculture, Horticulture, Forestry, Food, Nutrition and Consumer Sciences*. Available at: https://www.qaa.ac.uk/docs/qaa/subject-benchmark-statements/subject-benchmark-statement-agriculture-horticulture-forestry-food-nutrition-and-consumer-sciences.pdf?sfvrsn=28f2c881_7 (accessed 7 June 2021).

Riis, J., McFadden, B.R. and Collins, K. (2019) Thinking critically about nutrition, *Today's Dietitian*, 21, 36.

Ruben, A.M. (2016) How to read a scientific paper. Available at: https://www.sciencemag.org/careers/2016/01/how-read-scientific-paper (accessed 7 June 2021).

Tomlin, G. and Borgetto, B. (2011) Research pyramid: a new evidence-based practice model for occupational therapy, *American Journal of Occupational Therapy*, 65: 189–96.

5 Group work

Overview and outline

Most degrees will include some form of group work, whether that is in tutorials and seminars, laboratory practicals or a group assessment. Working in a group or team is an important skill that you will need to develop at university, but it will also be essential in your future career. It is important you know how to be a good team member and work harmoniously with others. This chapter will outline the skills you will acquire, make suggestions for how to get off to a good start, consider the different roles people can play in teams and look at troubleshooting common problems.

We know many of you are likely to actively dislike group work and would generally prefer to work on your own. However, there are some advantages to working in a group. It allows you to tackle bigger problems than you could on your own. It helps you to incorporate different viewpoints and ways of thinking. It might be good to chat with other people in your class. Dare we say it, but group work might even be fun! Group work can also help you develop a whole host of transferable skills and include the sorts of skills that employers will be looking for. Therefore you may want to ensure you can describe these skills in your personal statement.

What skills will teamwork help you develop?

These skills are likely to include the following.

- Communication
- Cooperation
- Decision making
- Delegating
- Feedback
- Leadership
- Listening
- Organisation

Who is in the group?

Sometimes you may pick your own groups but at other times the groups may be chosen for you. This might seem unfair but remember that when you start work you will not be able to choose who is in your team, so it is important to think about how to get the best out of any team situation. If you work with the same people all the time you might find that you all have a similar skill set. But working with other class members will give you the opportunity to learn from other people and their experiences. Be careful about making a group too large as it can be difficult to co-ordinate and to know who is doing what.

Setting ground rules

Before you get started it is important to consider setting a few ground rules. This can help ensure everyone is on the same page before you get deeper into the project. For example, common rules might include:

- Attendance and turning up to meetings
- Being on time
- Deciding who will chair
- Agreeing who will take notes
- Confidentiality
- Putting away mobiles
- Being respectful to each other and different opinions

Planning your group work

Getting started on a group project can always be a bit tricky, so consider the following ideas to get going:

1 If you don't already know each other, spend some time introducing your-selves.
2 You may want to set some guidelines about how you want to work together.
3 You might want to appoint a leader or a chairperson.
4 See if someone can offer to take notes of the meeting; though you might want to take turns to do this.
5 Check you all understand the project brief in the same way.
6 Brainstorming is a great way for everyone to throw in their own ideas. Make it clear that no idea is a bad one in order to encourage everyone to participate before you decide which direction you want to take the project.

7 Consider if the project can be broken down into smaller chunks that you could distribute between you.

8 Check that everyone knows what they are doing and when it needs to be completed by.

9 Consider how will you communicate between meetings; is everyone happy to share their university email address?

10 Organise your next meeting; this might be easier said than done particularly if you all have different timetables, but it is important to fix a date in the diary. Meetings don't always have to be in person; you could use Skype or Zoom if that is easier.

Forming, storming, norming, performing and adjourning

You may have come across Tuckman's (1965) group development model. This model describes the theoretical phases that a team must go through to develop as a cohesive group that can work together effectively and overcome obstacles to produce an end product. These phases are described in Table 5.1.

Table 5.1 Forming, storming, norming, performing and adjourning

Phases	Description
Forming	This is the part where you form or pick the team, work out who is who, set any ground rules and start to become orientated with the project. It might also be the phase where everyone is a bit quiet and polite as you start to establish your roles.
Storming	At this point the goals are probably clearer, and you can start to establish some structure. It can be a tricky phase as you discover that you may have different ways of working and there could be the potential for conflict if you are not careful.
Norming	By this phase it is likely you have all worked out your roles, have accepted one another and have a known routine as you move towards your group objective.
Performing	This is the productive stage where by now you have created a friendly and creative environment, you can be strategic with a common focus and perform well together to complete your task.
Adjourning	Once the project is complete this might be the end of the group and you might even be sad to finish. But if you all get along well there is no reason why you cannot continue as a study group.

(Based on: Tuckman 1965)

You may have come across other variations on this model that include phases such as re-norming and transforming. You may move through some of these phases faster than others. In fact, you may not even go through these phases at all; every group is different. But understanding the phases that groups usually work through can help you understand more about group dynamics to help your group avoid common pitfalls and become more effective.

Team roles

There are numerous descriptions of different types of roles for team members within any group. Sometimes three key roles are described: Technical, Functional and Team Player. Sometimes four team role types are listed: Leader, Facilitator, Coach or Member. But probably the most well established are the nine team roles described by Belbin (1981); see Table 5.2. Members of your group

Table 5.2   Team roles

Role	Advantages	Disadvantages
1. Resource Investigator	Outgoing, brings the ideas and has an inquisitive nature	Might be overoptimistic or unrealistic
2. Plant	Inventive and thinks outside the box	Can be preoccupied and lack attention to detail
3. Co-ordinator	Shows leadership and distributes work, clarifies goals	Might delegate own jobs to others
4. Team Worker	Sensitive and diplomatic to all	Can have difficulties making decisions and will avoid confrontation
5. Shaper	Brings the energy and responds to barriers and deadlines	Has the potential to offend or hurt people's feelings
6. Specialist	Has the in-depth knowledge and technical skills	Can have a narrow viewpoint and will focus on the technicalities
7. Monitor-Evaluator	Calm and strategic with a good overview	May lack drive and can be negative
8. Implementer	Reliable and gets things done	Can be too rigid
9. Completer Finisher	Good attention to detail and refines work	Could be perfectionist and not share work

(Based on: Belbin 1981; University of Portsmouth 2021)

may have a natural affinity with the behaviours associated with some of the particular roles described. Understanding how individuals work can help ease communication within the group and help you work together effectively.

Do you recognise yourself in any of these roles? Could you share these roles out amongst your team? Belbin (1981) thought that good teams should have a balance of these roles and that imbalances would cause potential issues. Other research (Pritchard and Stanton 1991) has also confirmed that mixed teams do appear to work more effectively than teams where there is a large imbalance of roles. However, perhaps you see yourself in a number of these roles; in fact there may be overlap between some of the roles listed here. Perhaps not all the roles are required for your project. And let's not forget this model was developed with business management teams in mind rather than university students. Awareness of these roles, and the advantages and disadvantages associated with them, is useful and it may be helpful in understanding how different people work, but don't let it entirely define your contribution to the group project.

What makes effective teamwork?

Being organised – keep up to date with your work, know what has been done, what you are doing and what needs to be done next. Make notes and report back to each other. Being organised will save lots of time in the long run.

Listening – take time to listen to each other and value each other's opinions.

Set deadlines – not just for the final piece of work but set small tasks and targets for each of the team members. Create a timeline and try to stick to these deadlines to avoid letting the work slip.

Keep communication channels open – communicating clearly at meetings is important but also decide how best to communicate outside of meetings too. Use the group's preferred method of communication, whether that is by email or WhatsApp.

Encourage each other – some people may need some encouragement to contribute. Take turns to speak, giving everyone an opportunity and ensuring everyone is comfortable.

Delegate – it's important that everyone feels involved and can contribute, so don't dominate the project, share out the roles and ensure everyone feels part of the team.

Delegating

It can be very easy to think it would be easier just to do all the work yourself, but that isn't what teamwork is about. Sharing out the tasks will not only lighten your workload but will also help to keep everyone involved and feel part of the group. It is important that everyone feels like they are a valued team member and delegating actually encourages teamwork (Flores-Fillol et al. 2017). But it can be hard to delegate if you are not used to doing so.

The first thing is to make a list of tasks that need to be completed. Table 5.3 gives an example of a topic that has been broken down into manageable chunks that would need completing if you were working on a group presentation about vegetarianism. Using this example, you can understand how any project can be broken down into separate chunks (or tasks) that different team members can then take responsibility for.

Table 5.3   Example of tasks that need researching for a group presentation on vegetarianism

Vegetarian diet talk task	Who
✓ Definition of vegetarianism	
✓ Types of vegetarianism	
✓ Potential health benefits	
✓ Potential health concerns	
✓ Nutrients of note	
✓ Role for fortified food	
✓ Vegetarian food models	
✓ Conclusions – all to agree at next meeting	

Each person can be assigned to a different task, though some may need to be shared. Make sure someone keeps a note of who is doing what. Although most people will volunteer, there may be times when you need to allocate tasks to ensure all aspects are covered; make sure to do this in a fair and sympathetic manner. Do allow time in your meetings for everyone to feedback on what they have found and check you are all on track; some members of the team may need more support than others. If you are doing a piece of work like a poster, you might also want to make sure someone is given the responsibility of having general oversight to ensure the style looks consistent when everything is brought together. If you are doing a presentation you should factor in time for a rehearsal.

Troubleshooting

- Try not to do all the work yourself, remember it is a group project so try to share the workload fairly.
- Always be respectful of the opinions of others – even if they are very different from your own.

- If one or two people dominate the discussions, try to involve others in the group and hear their viewpoints. If you haven't done so already, you may need to appoint a chairperson to help facilities discussions.
- Does your group include some 'free loaders'? It might be that they are struggling and find the work difficult; perhaps they just need more help to understand the assignment. It is possible that they have lots of other commitments, so perhaps the group can be flexible with meeting times, etc. If it is that they are simply not bothered, try talking to them about it and explain why it is important to you. If one team member is consistently absent it might be worth discussing this with the lecturer. If you are the one who is always missing meetings, it is probably a good idea to contact the lecturer to explain why.
- Some people may dominate the meeting. Perhaps you can try and negate this by having different people chair the meeting each time. If you have particularly loud people in the group, perhaps ask everyone to write down their ideas and then go round the group and share, rather than just shouting your views out loud.
- Organising meetings can be difficult, particularly if you are taking different modules and have timetabling conflicts. Perhaps you could organise a doodle poll to work out the best time for everyone to meet?
- Sometimes there will be personality clashes. Although this may be difficult to avoid you can ensure that you all behave in a professional manner at all times – just as you would in a workplace. You don't have to be friends outside of the group work, but you do want to get the job done without arguments. Remember to negotiate and compromise. These are important skills to have and develop.
- If your group starts to lose focus, remember what it is you are trying to achieve. Break the work down into smaller tasks that can be ticked off as you complete them and get closer to your end goal.
- Avoid negativity and try to look for the positive in everyone's contribution. Instead of saying something is wrong, could you turn it into a question? Avoid negative body language too, crossing your arms and staring might not give the impression you are keen to be involved.
- Ensuring good communication is going to be key in any group or team. People want to feel their contributions are valued and may worry if they miss things. Writing up notes from the meetings and sharing them with the group can help with this, as well as regular updates and progress reports, which can also help smooth the path to completion.

Group tutorials

Whilst you may have some personal tutorials you may also be expected to attend and contribute to group tutorials. Group tutorials are essential for further developing important skills including communication and critical thinking. These tutorials will probably also help deepen your subject knowledge and understanding.

Tutorials are usually organised in small groups and are therefore less formal than lectures. They usually relate to the modules you are taking and may involve discussions and related activities, such as going over assessments, receiving or providing feedback, practice exam papers, even pastoral and wellbeing advice. Formats of tutorials may vary and this will depend on the lecturer.

Do make sure that you carry out adequate preparation for a tutorial. First of all, you need to know what the tutorial is about. If you have been asked to read or prepare something, do ensure you allow time in your schedule to do this. Tutorials present an opportunity to discuss your work with an academic and with other students, so it is a good way to check your understanding of the subject and develop it further. You may even want to prepare some questions that you would like to ask beforehand.

Listen to what the lecturer and other students are saying. You may not always agree with what is being said, and that is fine. If you want to disagree, stay calm and try to present facts related to your viewpoint. If you don't understand something, then say so. You will probably find that there are others in the group who are feeling the same and will be relieved that others are in the same position. Do be sensitive to others and allow them to present their viewpoints even if they are different to yours. Being respectful to everyone is essential in tutorial situations.

Seminars

Seminars are another situation where you might find yourself working in a smaller group. Often seminars are arranged to discuss a topic or a journal paper that links to your lectures. The seminar may start with a short presentation, either by the lecturer or sometimes a student, followed by questions and discussions. Again, it is worth making sure you prepare well for a seminar by ensuring you have read the relevant paper and perhaps highlighted relevant parts, made notes on your opinions, done a critique of the paper or noted any questions you would like to ask. If you don't understand something don't be afraid to say so; staff will always be supportive, especially if you can show you have done the reading and want to try and understand it further.

To get the most out of a seminar, see it as another learning opportunity and try to participate. As with tutorials, do make sure you listen to other students, respect their opinions and be positive about the contributions of others even if you don't agree. Perhaps instead of saying 'I disagree' this could be phrased as 'I can see your point but have you considered ...'. Discussion is good and you may even change your mind several times during the discussion if you are open to the views of others.

If you are shy, try to find ways to build your own confidence, such as planning ahead and writing down any comments you would like to make. Don't assume everyone else in the room knows more about the subject than you; most of your peers are likely to be feeling the same. But seminars should be a supportive environment where you can help each other to explore a subject and build confidence in a manageable way. You will probably find that the more you say, the easier it gets. If you are finding it hard to get a word into the discussion, just raise your hand to show you would like to contribute. If you don't already know the other students, try to make a friend at each seminar, this might also help make the seminar experience feel less awkward.

If you are a more confident person, try not to dominate the discussion yourself but make sure everyone gets an opportunity to express their views. Try to be supportive of people who may find this more challenging.

Without clock watching, do keep an eye on time; for example if you have four questions to answer, you don't want to spend most of the time debating the first question and then run out of time before you get to consider the other questions. It might even be worth agreeing how long you want to spend on each question at the start. It is also worth writing some notes as you go along so you don't forget what you have agreed or learnt earlier in the discussions.

At the end of the seminar, try to reflect on what you have learnt and write down a summary of the key notes. This might really help with revision later.

Never be tempted to miss your seminars: they can be one of the best ways for finding out more about your subject in depth and this will really help with your understanding and learning.

Laboratory practicals

As part of your nutrition and or dietetics degree you are likely to have several laboratory practicals. On some occasions you may work alone, but probably in most cases you will work with a partner or in threes. Being in the lab is a great opportunity to develop some specific research techniques, so do make sure everybody gets the opportunity to contribute to the experiment, and practise the particular method being taught. Whether you are pipetting, titrating or streaking microbiology plates, you will only get better with practice so ensure you each take turns to have a go.

Check how group work will be marked

For some assignments, lecturers will just award a group mark. Others may award individual marks within the group. It is not always clear if the work has been evenly spread in a group project so some lecturers may ask you to write up your contribution to the project or even ask you to rate each other's performance.

Some universities, but not all, give marks for participation in tutorials and seminars so do check if this is the case. If this is the case, then make sure you attend and are prepared and ready to participate.

You should also check what levels of collaboration will be permitted for any work submitted. For some group work you may collect data together but write individual reports; for example this is common when it comes to laboratory work. For other work you may just give one presentation or write one report on behalf of the whole group. So check you know what is expected of you to avoid the risk of being penalised for collusion.

Other places you can develop your teamwork skills

Group assessments are not the only places where you can develop your teamwork skills. You might be part of a sports team or on the committee of a student society; charity work and part-time employment will also give you opportunities to work as part of a team. So do consider these options when looking for examples of experience of teamwork when putting your CV together or completing any application forms.

Summary

Group work can be challenging but it can also be rewarding and help you develop many useful transferable skills. You may now understand the importance of setting ground rules and planning the work carefully as you negotiate different phases of group development. You may appreciate the different roles that people may take on to form an effective team, and how these roles and different tasks can be shared out amongst the group. Hopefully you will also have seen how to avoid common pitfalls in order to work successfully together as a group, whether that is in a tutorial and seminar situation, laboratory practical or for assessments.

Reflective questions

- What role/s are you most comfortable with when participating in group work?
- Are there skills you would like to develop further? For example, would you volunteer to be the team leader next time you need to participate in group work?
- How can you ensure everyone in your team participates?

Suggested further reading

Belbin, M. (2021) The nine Belbin team roles. Available at: https://www.belbin.com/about/belbin-team-roles/
Levin, P. (2004) *Successful Team Work*. London: Open University Press.

References

Belbin, M. (1981) *Management Teams*. London: Heinemann.

Flores-Fillol, R., Iranzo, S. and Mane, F. (2017) Teamwork and the delegation of decisions within the firm, *International Journal of Industrial Organization*, 52: 1–29.

Prichard, J.S. and Stanton, N.A. (1999) Testing Belbin's team role theory of effective groups, *Journal of Management Development*, 18(8): 652–65.

Tuckman, B.W. (1965) Developmental sequence in small groups, *Psychological Bulletin*, 65: 384–99.

University of Portsmouth (2021) Help and advice. Available at: https://www.port.ac.uk/student-life/help-and-advice/study-skills/working-in-groups/allocating-and-developing-team-roles (accessed 26 March 2021).

6 Oral and poster presentations

Overview and outline

It is highly likely that at some point during your degree you will be asked to do a presentation. This might be an oral presentation or a poster presentation, though it is likely you will get the opportunity to do both during your time at university. This chapter will outline what you need to consider when preparing for an oral or a poster presentation to ensure you can present your information clearly and become a confident public speaker.

Oral presentations

Speaking

At the start of any presentation, make sure you introduce yourself clearly, give your name and also the title of your talk. Ensure that you are speaking loudly enough for all your audience to hear you, even if they are sitting at the back of the room. If you are in a lecture room you may need to stay close to the microphone for everyone to be able to hear you, so try not to do too much moving around. You might be given a clip-on microphone, which will allow you more freedom; even so, try not to do too much pacing up and down.

Try to talk slowly and clearly. You will probably need to speak slightly more slowly than you normally would, and this might feel unnatural at first, but it will help your audience understand what you are saying. Try recording yourself and listening back; do you gabble or change speeds, and could you slow this down if you needed to?

Try to look at your audience, even if you need to read some of your notes, do ensure you look up regularly and make eye contact with the people in the room. We know some people say you should imagine the audience in their underwear; however, we think this could be more off-putting, and so prefer to focus on the material being presented rather than the audience. But you can always look for the 'nodders'; there are bound to be some people in the audience who nod as they listen, we always find it very reassuring to see people who are nodding at what we are saying.

Think about your body language. Do you pace up and down or do you stand rigidly still? What do you do with your hands while you are talking? If you can, it is useful to video yourself rehearsing your presentation, you might be surprised how much you fidget whilst you are talking. It is good to make eye contact with your audience; it is also good to smile and be enthusiastic about your presentation too.

Slides

For some oral presentations you will also need to prepare some slides to accompany the talk. PowerPoint is frequently used in universities but other packages, including Prezi, may also be used.

When you are creating your slides, you should ensure you make good use of the visual material. Think about your use of colour. Whilst you want the slides to be bright and interesting, you don't want too many clashing colours as this could make them difficult for some people to read. You should think about the best colour scheme that looks interesting and professional but is also clear.

Do make sure the text is legible and can be read from a distance. Bullet points are usually better than long passages of text and, in fact, you should avoid text-heavy slides; you don't want to end up just reading your slides. If you can include a relevant figure, graph or table then you should do so, as often this could explain your point better than text alone. Two examples of slides are shown in Fig. 6.1, one is text heavy and the other contains the same information but is better presented and more eye catching (though bear in mind the image is in black and white here).

It is fine to include some pictures or clip art but don't add too many images. Likewise, don't overdo the animations and special effects; too many slides whooshing and appearing all over the place might distract the audience from your more serious points.

Figure 6.1 Examples of two slides showing the same information

Good Sources of Calcium

There are many good food sources of calcium and these include the dairy products such as milk, yoghurt and cheese. However, calcium is also available in some non-dairy foods. Non dairy sources of calcium include leafy green vegetables and almonds. Some vegan foods such as soya drinks are also fortified with calcium.

Good Sources of Calcium

Dairy products:
 – Milk
 – Cheese
 – Yoghurt

Vegan options
 – Almonds
 – Green leafy vegetables
 – Soya drinks fortified with calcium

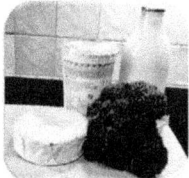

You should also make sure your slides are referenced appropriately. It is surprising how many students know how to reference an essay correctly but don't remember to use references on their presentation sides.

Also, don't have too many slides; you don't want to be constantly flicking through slides and you want to ensure the audience have enough time to read them. A rough guideline would be ten slides for a 10-minute presentation; so no more than one a minute.

Visual aids

Slides are not the only visual materials you can incorporate. Other ideas for visual aids that you could use include:

- Examples of a product
- Flip chart
- Handouts
- Pictures/photos
- Samples
- Short video
- Whiteboard

Feel free to use the visual aids that are most appropriate for your talk, but do rehearse with them and ensure they don't get in the way of delivery of the key content of the talk. If you are using anything such as videos, do check beforehand that your links work.

Organisation and planning

A good talk is one that is planned well in advance. We all know people who are naturally gifted speakers, but they still need to ensure they have good content to rely on.

Think about the structure of your talk. Could you arrange your content so that it tells a story or starts with a question and then gives more detail before circling back to answer the original question? Or, in some cases, you could follow the basic structure of a report: introduction, methods, results, discussion, conclusion; though this might depend on the brief you were given for your presentation.

Plan what you need to convey on each slide, use headings, and then go back and add the details. Consider what are the main points you need to convey? It might be tempting to pack your talk with lots of details, but be careful you don't lose sight of your key arguments or points; clarity is key.

Ensure the content of your talk is scientifically sound. When talking about diet and nutrition it is easy to become quite anecdotal, but you should avoid this and guarantee your information is evidence based. It is important to have good quality references, including journal papers, and try to put the research into context to show your understanding.

Notes

Many students like to start with a full script of the talk written out, but the danger here is that you simply read the entire talk. Usually it is better if you can just write key notes or prompts. Some people like to put the prompts on the slides themselves, but be careful you don't just end up reading the slides, remember the audience can do that themselves.

Key notes and or bullet points, whether on paper or on flash cards, can remind you what you need to say but will have the advantage that they can enable a more fluid and natural style of presentation.

For more complicated parts where you need to be entirely accurate, or if you have a real concern that you might go blank, you can write fuller notes. However, do ensure you remember to look up at the audience, and try to vary the tone of your voice; don't just read monotonously with your head down.

You might worry about losing your place in your notes, but there are simple ways to prevent this. You could organise your notes so they correspond to each individual slide and number them as such, or use highlighter pens to pick out the key points, and then you can quickly identify these points as and when you need them. Also make sure the font and line spacing are large enough on your notes so that you can find the right place easily.

Timing

Do a practice run through of your talk and time it to make sure it is not too long or not too short. You could record your talk so you can hear yourself speaking; you may find that you speak faster than you think you do, so check if you need to slow down or add another point of discussion. If you overrun on time the lecturer may stop you and you may not get to conclude your talk. Check the time allowed for your talk and time for questions; is the question time included in your talk time or given separately? Generally it is better to be a minute too short than too long, as this is easier to adjust the programme around with more time for questions or longer breaks. However, if your talk is too short it may look like you needed to do more research, so do try to use the allocated time wisely.

If there are any complicated words or chemical names in your talk that you are not sure how to pronounce, you can check on Google by typing in 'how do you pronounce ...' and then you can practise them. Try not to draw attention to these words or highlight them during the talk; for example, never say 'I don't know how to pronounce this but ...' in most cases if you just say the word with confidence, no one will notice a thing. We are strong believers in this anonymous quote: *'Never make fun of someone if they mispronounce a word. It means they learned it by reading.'*

At the end of your talk

It is always good to have a strong closing statement or summary of the talk. Never just finish with 'that's it'. Make it clear you are coming to the end of your talk by using phrases such as 'And finally ...' or 'In conclusion ...' or even ultimately 'Thank you for your attention'. Smile, then you can invite the audience to ask questions.

Be ready to answer questions

It is highly likely there will be time for questions at the end of your talk. Try to think in advance about what questions you might be asked, so you can consider how you might answer them. Obviously, you cannot pre-empt all questions, so take your time to think about the question that was asked. If you are not sure you understand the question, ask the speaker to repeat the question or clarify. If you really don't know (and you cannot be expected to know everything) you can say something like 'that's a really good question', then answer the parts you do know and add something along the lines of 'I would need to do more research to be able to fully answer that'. It is better to be honest than say something that may be incorrect.

On the day

Make sure you have a copy of your slides and you know where the venue for your presentation is. You may have had to submit the slides before the session or you may be expected to bring them on a USB stick or flash drive. It's also a good idea to email them to yourself in the event you need a backup. Get to the room early so you are not flustered and can choose where to sit. If you are not familiar with the room it will also give you time to work out where you should stand to give your presentation. Check you have your notes or cards to hand if you need them, and you can read over them whilst you wait for the session to start. You might want to have a bottle of water handy in case your mouth gets a little dry. Think calm and confident and you've got this!

Poster presentations

In the field of nutrition and dietetics there are two types of poster that you may be asked to create. One is a campaign or advertising poster and the other is an academic conference-style poster. Do check which type of poster is expected and will be the most appropriate for the sort of assignment you are working on.

Campaign poster

In modules related to health promotion or public health you might be asked to create a poster to promote or advertise a campaign. Think for example of a 'stop smoking' poster or a 'Five a Day' campaign aimed at the general public. This is an assignment where you can really be as creative as you like. The poster should:

- Be bright and clear
- Have a striking image or photo

- Contain a simple but effective message or slogan
- Have limited amounts of text.

Exposure to health promotion messages through poster campaigns by the general public is generally passive, therefore the main aim of this style of poster is to be eye catching and attention grabbing, particularly since the posters need to compete with other marketing adverts. However, studies have shown that mass media campaigns can have positive effects when it comes to changing population health behaviours (Wakefield et al. 2010) so the message on the poster is important to get right; make it catchy and memorable. The poster should speak for itself and be quick to understand without any further context or background information. Some good examples of this sort of poster can probably be found on public transport in most towns, or online take a look at government campaigns such as Change 4 Life.

Academic poster

Academic posters are commonly presented at conferences and you may even have seen a few displayed on the notice boards in your university department. These tend to be very focused and specific, have more text and are aimed at an academic audience.

Academic posters can be printed out on paper, usually size A1 or A0, and displayed on a board. Or posters can be electronic and displayed on a screen. In fact, we have even seen posters printed on material to make them easier to travel with. In all cases, the general principles are the same.

Poster dimensions

Check what size your poster should be. This should be in the assessment details or the conference information. As previously stated, posters for conferences are usually A1 or A0. A normal piece of paper, such as the ruled lined paper you might put in a folder, is considered A4. The dimensions of the other papers sizes are outlined below in Table 6.1.

Table 6.1 Paper sizes

Paper size	Equivalent number of pieces of A4	Dimensions (mm)
A4	1	210 x 297
A3	2	297 x 420
A2	4	420 x 594
A1	8	594 x 841
A0	16	841 x 1189

Most printers only print A4 or A3, so if you are required to print a larger poster you may need to go to your university print shop to do so. Poster printing can be quite costly, especially if you get it laminated. So check that you do actually need to print it. If the poster is for an assessment, some departments will get them printed for you. But often these days the poster may be displayed electronically so it is not necessary to get the poster printed at all.

Text

Although an academic poster will have more text than a campaign poster, you still want to reduce the amount of text where possible. It needs to be eye catching and easy to read, not just a report pasted onto a poster template. Try to include bullet points, tables, graphs or figures, as these can highlight the main points and can be read quickly. Although the word count may depend on the topic or assignment a rough guide is usually around 400 words, which is much less than an essay or report. Do make sure you are consistent with the font and size of the print you use. All headings should be the same size, likewise all the text, as this will make the poster look neater. Paragraphs can be justified to the left or fully justified so both the left and right margins are straight. Also think about line spacing; double spaced is usually easier to read, but 1.5 might work if you have space constraints.

Organisation

Many people use PowerPoint to create their poster, working on A4 which is then enlarged when printed onto A1 or A0.

Check the dimensions required and which page orientation your poster should be in, i.e. portrait or landscape?

Figure 6.2 Portrait or landscape

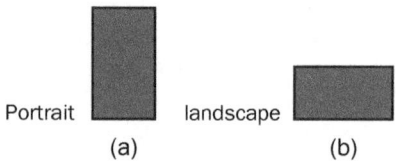

Make sure your title is clear and at the top of the poster. You should also ensure your name is visible and you may also want to add your university affiliation here too.

It usually best to present the information in blocks. If you are presenting an experiment or a study for example you might organise this into the following sections:

- Background
- Aim
- Methods

- Results
- Discussion
- Conclusion
- References

Examples of templates for posters using this style of organisation in both portrait and landscape orientation can be seen in Fig. 6.3 and Fig. 6.4. Relevant images can also be included in addition to the graphs and tables.

Figure 6.3 Example of a poster template in portrait orientation

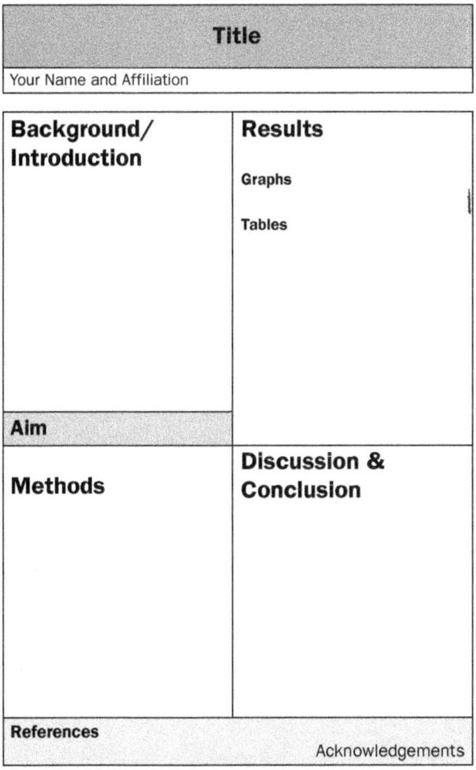

The material

Posters are usually aimed at an academic audience in a specialist subject field so you will need to ensure the content is accurate and evidence based. This also means you probably do not need to provide too much basic background material, and it is absolutely fine to use technical terms; however, you should check who the audience will be as, if the audience is more general, you may want to ensure you provide sufficient explanations.

Figure 6.4 Example of a poster template in landscape orientation

Title	Names	Affiliations
Aim **Background/ Introduction**	**Methods**	**Results continued** Table
	Results Graph	**Conclusion** **References**
Acknowledgements		

Images

Do make sure any images you use are relevant to the material being presented, and not just to make the poster look pretty. Pictures or diagrams should have numbers, titles and references if appropriate too. Take care with making images too big as they can become pixelated if the image is not of high enough resolution. It is also easy to over-stretch an image too high or wide; what looks fine on a computer screen or on A4 paper can look quite different when printed out on A0.

Tables are another way of presenting information in a clear format, so ensure they are relatively simple and easy to read. Check the font and line spacing are large enough so the table is clear. Sometimes tables look better if the contents are centred, particularly if you are presenting numbers; however, if your tables include text then justified to the left is probably neater. Also think about the lines on the table, do you need a complete grid?

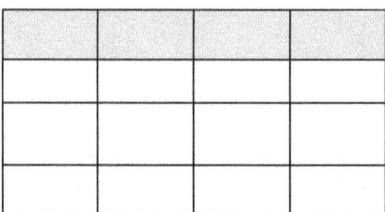

Or could you just include the horizontal lines and remove the vertical lines for further clarity or to highlight the flow of data?

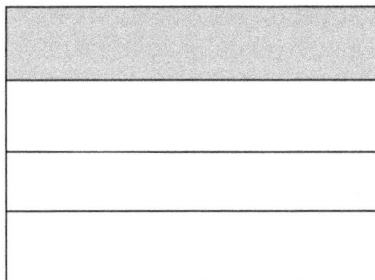

Graphs are an excellent way of conveying information or results clearly. First, make sure you have drawn the right sort of graph (e.g. bar chart, scatter graph, pie chart, etc.), not just the most colourful one. (explained in chapter 3) You do not need to keep to the colours that the chart wizard automatically created; you can change the colours so they are in keeping with the colour scheme of the rest of the poster. Make sure your graph is labelled fully with axis titles, units for the data and keys, as you would in any report.

Designs and colour cschemes

You want your poster to stand out, but you don't want to overdo it so there are clashing colours which are an eyesore. Think about the colour of the text that will make for easy reading; e.g. yellow text on a white background will be difficult to see from a distance, whereas black text is usually easier to read. Choose a colour scheme based on two or three complementary colours or even shades of the same colour. Try to tie in the colour of the background, headings and text with the images and graphs you have included too.

Proofreading

Finally, remember to proofread your work carefully. Mistakes can really stand out when they are printed large on A0 and displayed on the wall. If you can get someone else to proofread the poster too, that would be a good idea, as they just might notice something that you did not.

Presenting your poster

On the day of your presentation, make sure your poster is in the right place at the right time. You will probably be allocated a board or a station where your poster will be displayed. If you are doing a paper poster you may need to bring with you drawing pins, sticky tack or sticky strips; although most conference organisers will provide these. In some cases, you will be asked to stand by your poster and just answer any questions that people viewing the posters may have. However, sometimes you are expected to give a short oral presentation next to your poster. Usually this would be for no more than 5 minutes plus time for questions. You can have notes or flash cards for the oral presentation but, in most cases, you can use the poster itself to act as reminder prompts for what you need to say. Speak clearly and to the audience (not to the poster). Feel free to point to relevant parts of the poster such as an important graph or key data. Just as you would if you were doing an oral presentation, let the audience know when you are coming to the end of your talk using a phrase such as 'in conclusion ...' Then thank the audience for listening and ask if they have any questions. Afterwards, don't take your poster down too quickly as other people may still be looking at the posters; but you may have to remove it within a certain time frame, particularly if there is another poster session starting right after yours.

Summary

Presentations can be either oral presentations or poster presentations; and posters can be campaign posters or academic posters. This chapter has explained the different types of presentations and how you can prepare your materials, whether they are slides or a poster, to ensure your message is conveyed clearly, is well presented and eye-catching. You should also be able to think about how you communicate to your audience verbally and with visual aids. Be prepared to speak clearly, look confident and be ready to answer questions. And lastly, remember to proofread and practise!

Reflective questions

- Think of a good talk or poster that you have seen recently. What stood out to you?
- Could you record yourself rehearsing a presentation and then watch it back to identify things you could do differently?
- When you have given a presentation, what feedback have you received from the audience?

Suggested further reading

Levin, P. and Topping, G. (2006) *Perfect Presentations*. Maidenhead: Open University Press.

Public Health England (n.d.) *Change 4 Life* resources. Available at: https://campaignresources.phe.gov.uk/resources/campaigns/17-change4life/resources (for some examples of campaign posters and leaflets).

Reference

Wakefield, M.A., Loken, B. and Hornik, R.C. (2010) Use of mass media campaigns to change health behaviour, *The Lancet*, 376: 1261–71. https://doi.org/10.1016/S0140-6736(10)60809-4

7 Preparing for exams

Overview and outline

Love them or loathe them, and we are guessing most of you will loathe them, all university courses will include at least one exam. This chapter will help you think about the best ways to study and will help you to get organised to prepare for your exams through active revision and practice. It will also remind you to take care of yourself, so you are able to do your best on the day.

Introduction

Although exams have been criticised for being outdated tests of memory, they can encourage learning and are a good way of assessing depth and breadth of knowledge. A well-designed exam can help you identify your strengths and weaknesses, and can also assess your synthesis of information and even the application of that knowledge to real-world situations (Van Bergen and Lane 2016). Whatever your views on exams, it is likely that, at some point during your degree, you will need to sit one. With proper preparation and good revision skills, you can put yourself in the best position to perform well and do your absolute best whilst keeping a healthy perspective.

Advantages

There are some advantages to exams. For a start, you won't be expected to give particularly lengthy answers. Nor will you have to write out long detailed reference lists. Exams often have a greater focus on breadth as opposed to depth. They are also a good way of encouraging you to retain information and reflect on what you have learnt. But, perhaps most importantly, exams offer you a chance to show what you know.

Revision

In order to do well in your exams, you want to feel confident going into that exam hall and the best way to do that is to ensure you have prepared adequately.

Be organised! If you plan ahead, and make sure you allow yourself enough time to put the work in, you will be more self-assured when you start that exam.

A revision plan or timetable is a good idea. Check how many exams you have and calculate how many days you have between now and the exam period. Make your timetable realistic and do allow times for breaks. However, don't spend too much time designing and colour coding your exam timetable, rather than just getting on with the process of revision.

Before you start, check you know what you will be examined on and then spend some time getting all your notes and relevant information together.

- Do you have all the material you need?
- Do you need to track down any lecture notes or journal papers?
- Is there an online learning platform for the module you are studying (e.g. Moodle, Blackboard etc.)?
- Is there a textbook that would also support your learning?
- Have you received any feedback on other work in the same module that you can reflect on?

As soon as possible you should check the style of the exam by looking at past papers. Is it an unseen exam or a revealed paper? On occasion you may even get an open book exam.

How many questions will there be, and what type of questions will be asked? Exam questions can take many forms, including multiple choice, short answers, long answers, essays, case studies, problem based or any combination of these.

Check how long the exam is; you can then work out how much time to allow yourself on each question.

For example, if you had a two-hour exam paper where 40 per cent of the marks were for short answer questions and 60 per cent of the marks were for two essay questions you might decide to plan accordingly:

- 45 minutes for the short answers
- 35 minutes for each essay question
- 5 minutes at the end for checking over your answers
- Total 120 minutes

It is also worth checking how many marks are allocated to each question; you may want to allow a longer time for those questions with more marks.

Most lecturers will provide copies and examples of past papers and the types of questions, but some universities may hold copies of the papers in the library or an online repository. Occasionally papers may be withheld, but the lecturer will nearly always provide examples in class of the sort of thing to expect in the actual exam.

Active revision

Make sure you leave enough time for revision. Although many studies have shown that it's not the total number of study hours that are important but study quality and preparedness (Cross et al. 2016), you still need to ensure you allow adequate amounts of time to do this. Revision should be an active process: very few people will get by simply reading their notes. Active revision could be practice tests and dry runs of exams or it could be writing and organising your notes. Listed below are some ideas to help you revise actively:

- Organise your notes into categories – file dividers or colour coding can help.
- Summarise and condense the information; some students like to put this information on flash cards. Flash cards can also conveniently fit in your pocket so you can read them at the bus stop or whilst doing other activities (just make sure you remove them from your pocket before you go into your exam!).
- Practise doing past papers. This gives you an opportunity to test what you know, acknowledge what you don't know and need to revisit, and work out the time required.
- Some students look at past papers to try and identify patterns in the questions that are asked. However, you should not rely on this approach, as lecturers regularly update the content of their lectures and so the exams will be updated to reflect that.
- Try writing out model answers or explain a concept to a friend; understanding can really help with memory.
- If you do need to remember specific entities or concepts, some people find mnemonics helpful. Mnemonics are memory aids that are particularly useful if you need to remember lists of things in a certain order. One such example of a mnemonic that we were taught many years ago at school, for taxonomy classifications in biology, that we can still remember today is as follows:
  - Kindly Put Coffee On For Guest Speaker
  - Kingdom, Phylum, Class, Order, Family, Genus, Species

  You can make your own up to remember key facts or even formulae.

- Test yourself or get others to test you. Testing is well known as being good for memory (Vaughn and Rawson 2011).
- Be as creative as you like, illustrating and colouring in your study notes may help you remember more.
- Audio cues can also be useful, record yourself reading your revision notes onto your phone and listen back to them later, for example whilst doing other activities such as cooking a meal.

Put your phone away and be honest with yourself: are you really focusing on your revision or are you trying to do two things at once? Although some people find listening to classical music helpful (Dosseville et al. 2012), watching TV at the same time as revising is probably not. It is also important to take regular breaks. So you could reward yourself for doing revision with a break to watch a short television programme or read a magazine, do some exercise or some other activity.

Don't procrastinate or put off your revision; if you can tell yourself to do just 10 minutes you might then find you get to a point where you can do a bit more. If you are bored, try using different techniques; you do not want the material and your revision to become stale.

Also consider if your environment is conducive to revision. Do you have space for your books and notes? Is the area well-lit, ventilated and quiet enough? Do you prefer to work in your room or the university library? Some people prefer to work in a setting that would be similar to that experienced in an exam hall (quiet and with an individual desk) to help them get in the right mind set and feel more relaxed and familiar with those conditions on the day.

We know many students work in part-time jobs, or have caring responsibilities, so make the most of short periods of time; for example, put your notes on a card that you can read in your breaks, waiting for the kettle to boil, or on the bus.

It's also worth considering your writing speed – we are all so used to using keyboards, will you struggle to write for two hours using pen and paper? It might be worth practising writing your exam answers in a time frame similar to that which you will have for the actual exam.

Different types of exams

As previously stated, exams can take many forms. Below you can find advice for multiple choice, short answer and essay-based exams:

Multiple choice

If your exam is multiple choice, read the instructions carefully and check the timing; how long will you have per question? Take a detailed look at the marking system. While multiple-choice exams may award marks for correct answers, some exams may use negative marks for wrong answers; if this is the case, guessing could result in a lower mark. However, if negative scoring is not used you have nothing to lose by guessing any questions you are not sure about.

Carefully scan the papers you have been given. Sometimes there is a separate answer sheet for multiple choice questions. You might be asked to write directly on the question sheet, circling your answer with a pen, or you might be asked to shade an oval or box shape with a pencil; if this is the case make sure any pencil lines stay within the box to ensure it can be read accurately by the scanner or computer that will be used to automate the marking. You may even be given an answer grid on which to provide your answers, in which case double check the question numbers as you go, as putting an answer in the wrong box could have a knock-on effect on any subsequent answers.

If you change your mind about an answer, and you are using pen, cross out the wrong answer and ensure it is clear which answer you want marked. If you are using the pencil shading system you will need to ensure you carefully erase the wrong answer and then add the new answer clearly marked.

With most exam papers you probably want to read all the questions through first, before starting to write. However, with multiple choice, particularly if there are many questions, you may want to get started straightaway.

If you don't know an answer, don't dwell on it; move on and then come back to it at the end.

Although this might sound obvious, do read the questions very carefully, some questions may have only one response, for example:

Question 1. Which vitamin is needed for the synthesis of proteins that are required for blood clotting?

i. Vitamin A
ii. Vitamin B1
iii. Vitamin B12
iv. Vitamin K

The question may be worded to ask you to pick a statement that is true; conversely, you have to choose a statement that is **not** true, so make sure you have carefully read and understood the question. Furthermore, some questions may ask for you to indicate **all** that are true or apply, in this case you would be required to tick more than one answer, for example:

Question 2. Which of the following foods would be good sources of folate for someone who eats a vegan diet?

a) spinach
b) brazil nuts
c) sardines
d) onion
e) broccoli
f) peas
g) fortified breakfast cereals

Once you have completed all the questions you should go back and attempt any unanswered questions then, if you still have time, look back through the test and double check your answers.

Short answer questions

Short answer questions are usually open ended in style and are a direct test of knowledge. They usually require you to be factual and succinct. As always, read the question carefully to check you understand what you are being asked; for example, are you expected to 'list', 'describe' or 'define' a specified concept? Alternatively, you may be asked to read a graph or perform a calculation; if it is the latter, ensure you clearly show all your workings out.

Although you may not want to write a plan for a short answer question, it might be helpful to jot down the key words that you want to ensure your answer contains. For example, it is very easy to describe osmosis without actually using the word 'osmosis', and this might affect the marks that are awarded.

You may need to draw a diagram or a graph. In such cases the examiner is not concerned with your artistic skills but will be looking for clear presentation (so make it large enough) and to see that it is clearly and neatly labelled.

Finally, remember:

- Make sure your writing is clear and legible.
- At the end, review your answers, check spellings, grammar and clarity.

Essay-based questions

When doing essay-based exams, first read the paper carefully to see how many essays you are expected to write. If there is a choice, you will need to decide which essay or essays you want to answer. It might sound obvious but, in most cases, you should choose the one you know the most about! If you are having trouble deciding between two essays, you might even want to do two quick essay plans to decide which one you know more about and have the greatest understanding of.

Essay plans

Consider doing an essay plan to get your thoughts in order. It will only take 5 minutes but will help you to write a well-organised essay and you will be less likely to leave out important facts. Your plan could be a simple list of key words or paragraph headings, or you could quickly draw a spider diagram. Fig. 7.1 provides an example of an exam essay question and a plan to answer it done in the form of a spider diagram. Note, this is just an example and by no means deemed to be the perfect answer; there are probably many points you could

Figure 7.1 Example of an essay plan in the style of a spider diagram

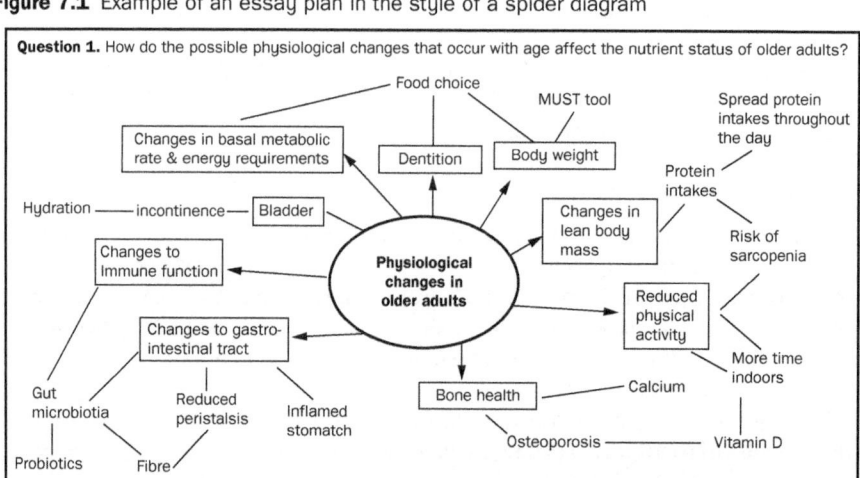

add or remove depending on the focus of your answer. Spider diagrams are also useful as part of your revision to help get your thoughts in order. In fact, essay plans in general are a good tool to use when revising. If you are reviewing past papers but do not have time to write a full practice essay, then write a plan for the essay you would write.

Remind yourself how much time you have for each question, leaving a few minutes at the end for proofreading.

Read the question through twice and ensure you know what you are being asked. Make sure you answer the question – don't just write everything you know on the subject; however, if all else fails do write something (anything) as you may be able to pick up a few marks here and there, and once you start writing you may begin to remember more points you could include. Before you finish, go back and re-read the original question, and make sure you haven't veered off topic. In particular, check that your final conclusion relates to the original question.

Referencing

In an exam you would not be expected to use a large number of references but do try to use them where possible. You would normally only be expected to remember the author's name and year of publication, e.g. (Garrow 2013). In exam conditions you wouldn't be expected to write a full reference list at the end. However, using some references can show your depth of knowledge, awareness of seminal publications and provide evidence that you have done further reading.

Structure

An essay that is well structured will flow well. Does your essay at least have a beginning, a middle and an end? You may have several sections so do use paragraph headings if it helps to keep your essay well organised.

Don't be afraid to use tables, graphs or diagrams; keep them neat, give them a title and labels as appropriate and do make sure you refer to them in the text.

Do not write out an essay and try learn it off by heart, as it is highly unlikely you will get the exact same question, and you need to be able to adapt your answer to the specific question you have been given.

Try to stick to your time plan. If you are running out of time and need to move on to the next essay, leave a space as you may be able to come back to it later.

At the end of the exam, read through your work carefully and check your spelling and grammar too.

All exam situations

Double check the date, time and location of your exams; although it is unlikely, sometimes timetables and details of rooms are changed, and you do not want to be in the wrong place or arrive at the wrong time.

Make sure you leave enough time to get to your exam. This is particularly important if you are a commuting student, as train cancellations and over-crowding on buses can add considerable time to your journey. Some universities have rules that they will not permit anyone to enter the exam hall once the exam has started or, in some cases, 30 minutes after the exam has begun; check your university's regulations.

Once in the exam room, try to make the most of your time there, and do not leave the exam room early. Imagine how you would feel if the answer suddenly came to you but you were outside the exam hall with the examination still in progress.

Likewise, do not risk wasting any of your exam writing time; it might seem obvious, but always go to the loo before the exam starts.

If you are entitled to extra time, ensure the person invigilating knows this; you don't want a big discussion about this in the exam hall. In some cases, you might be in a different location from other people or in an individual room so check this in advance too.

What if you go 'blank' in an exam?

First of all, take a deep breath. Then observe your breath, breathe in for a count of three and out for a count of three. Close your eyes if it helps. Take a sip of water. Then, when you are ready, take another look at the question. Write down some key words; this might have a calming effect but may also prompt your memory. Just writing something on the paper can be a good start: you can cross out or change it and add other information later. However, the ideal thing to do, if you think this might happen to you, is to work out a personal plan for dealing with this, long before you go into the exam room. For example, your plan might be, 'If I go blank I will do breathing exercises, then I will write out a list of the topics I have revised …' etc. You can then follow your plan if the need arises. Academic or wellbeing advisors at your university should be able to help you with this too.

On the day of the exam

Try to stay as relaxed as you can and consider the following list of actions:

- Check the time and location of the exam again
- Eat breakfast if possible
- Make sure you have plenty of time to get to the exam venue
- Ensure you have pens, pencils, rulers in a clear bag or pencil case
- Calculator: if it is required and you are permitted
- A bottle of water
- Ensure you have your student ID card

If it doesn't go to plan

First: don't catastrophise or blow it out of proportion; you may have done better than you think.

If you don't pass, you are usually given a resit and, in some cases, two resits. Take time to think about what you could do differently next time. Did you revise the wrong things or not use the time effectively? It is not always possible, but it is worth asking your lecturer if you can see your exam paper to see how it was marked and to discuss how to improve. This will help you understand what happened and identify what you need to work on.

If you went blank or felt stressed, make an appointment with a tutor, academic advisor or student counsellor, to try and work out a strategy for how to deal with this. Do this straight away rather than wait until the exam period when it might be more difficult to get an appointment.

Look after yourself

As a Nutrition and/or Dietetics student you will already know how important a healthy lifestyle is. However, as you approach your exams it is important that you check that you are putting this into practice. Make sure you find time to eat properly, take some exercise, such as yoga or a walk outside, and ensure you are getting enough sleep; this will all help you feel better and perform your best on the day.

Don't be afraid to ask for help. If you are worried, then talk to your tutor or a lecturer. In addition, most universities will have a student welfare officer, advisor or counsellor you can talk to, and together you can plan a strategy to help you manage.

Summary

Hopefully this chapter has helped you plan your revision and has provided some ideas for active revision, as well as made you aware of the different types of exams and exam questions. Appreciate the importance of making time to prepare and practise exam techniques and looking at past papers. In addition, and most importantly, remember to take care of yourself and ask for help if you need it.

Reflective questions

- What are your usual revision techniques?
- Is your revision 'active revision'?
- How do you plan to prepare yourself the night before and on the day of the exam?

Suggested further reading

Cazalet, C. (2015) *The Holy Grail of Exam Success: A Modern Strategy for Body and Brain*. Croydon: MLC Publishing.

NHS (2017) Tips on surviving exams. Available at: https://www.nhs.uk/conditions/stress-anxiety-depression/tips-on-surviving-exams/ (accessed 4 November 2021).

References

Cross, S., Whitelock, D. and Mittelmeier, J. (2016) Does the quality and quantity of exam revision impact on student satisfaction and performance in the exam itself? Perspectives from undergraduate distance learners, *EDULEARN16 Proceedings*, IATED Academy, 5052–61.

Dosseville, F., Laborde, S. and Scelles, N. (2012) Music during lectures: Will students learn better? *Learning and Individual Differences*, 22: 258–62.

Van Bergen, P. and Lane, R. (2016) Should we do away with exams altogether? No, but we need to rethink their design and purpose. *The Conversation*, available at: https://theconversation.com/should-we-do-away-with-exams-altogether-no-but-we-need-to-rethink-their-design-and-purpose-67647 (accessed 17 December 2020).

Vaughn, K.E. and Rawson, K.A. (2011) Diagnosing criterion-level effects on memory: what aspects of memory are enhanced by repeated retrieval? *Psychological Science*, 22: 1127–31. doi:10.1177/0956797611417724

8 Studying online

Overview and outline

Over recent years there has been increasing interest in online courses; however, the COVID-19 pandemic forced many universities to switch to online teaching in a relatively short amount of time. Students and lecturers had to learn and adapt to this new way of teaching, and though it was challenging at times, we all learnt huge amounts. There are now many courses, webinars and conferences that are hosted online and, in many cases, universities have decided to keep the elements of online learning that worked best to offer a blended learning approach (blended learning includes both online and in-person teaching). This chapter will outline some of what we have learnt about studying online so you can make the most of the opportunities that this method can bring.

Getting set up for online learning

It might sound obvious but if you are going to study online you will need access to a computer, up-to-date software and a good Wi-Fi connection. Whilst mobile phones might work for some aspects of online learning, it will certainly make it more challenging, and they are not necessarily suitable for all the platforms you will want to use. Most universities will have computer suites, many open 24 hours a day, but if you are wanting to study online you may be working from home. Many universities have laptops that can be taken out on loan or even schemes to help fund laptops so it is worth checking out what your university may be able to offer in this area.

If you are working from home think about the physical space where you are going to study. Can you find somewhere you will be comfortable? Although it might be tempting to work on your bed, or in front of the television, this won't help you stay focused; plus you will want to spend time in these areas when you want to relax. If you can, try to create an area that you can make your study area. Keep it clear from clutter and lay out everything you need. Try to reduce other distractions, including the TV and social media. You may spend quite a bit of time in this area so think about the desk and chair. Are they comfortable, are they the right height to protect your back, neck and wrists? It would be worth doing a 'healthy and safety' style workstation check to protect your health and ensure your desk and computer set-up does not cause discomfort later. Think about your posture, and make sure you take plenty of breaks for your eyes, as well as your spine. Keep the space neat and tidy. If you like something green around you, you can add a plant or anything that will make the space somewhere you will be happy and comfortable to work. Remember that, even though you are working online, you may still have lots of handouts or hard copies of papers. Use folders and boxes to keep these files neat and organised too.

Managing your time

The beauty of online studying is that in most cases you can work flexibly. Think about when you study best, are you a morning lark or a night owl? Regardless of personal preference, you may have other aspects of your life to consider; important considerations, such as family and work, may need to be accommodated first. So, plan a timetable that works for you and your life. Finding a routine can help give you structure to your day and this can help you stay on top of your work and meet your deadlines.

You do need to organise time for online learning. Just as you would have a timetable for classes taught on campus, you should ensure you put live lecture times in your diary or planner. However, you should also make sure you plan time for the asynchronous activities, such as catching up on a recorded lecture, reading set texts, watching video clips, etc. Otherwise, it is too easy to think you will do them later and then not get round to doing them at all.

A paper or online diary will be useful, or you can create your own planner showing each week of term and targets for each module. An example of a very simple term planner is shown in Table 8.1 but you can add as much detail or

Table 8.1 Example of a term planner

Autumn term	Module/Unit 1	Module/Unit 2	Deadlines
Week			
1			
2			
3			
4			
5			
Reading week/Half term			
7			
8			
9			
10			
Exam week			

Table 8.2 Assessment completion plan

Target date	Aim – to complete Measuring Energy Expenditure Report by 14 Feb (submission deadline 16th Feb)
1 February	Start: read and clarify the assignment details
2 February	Work out what information you need to gather, check the structure of the report
4 February	Complete the background reading and start the introduction
6 February	Write the methods section
9 February	Ensure you have the data and write up the results
11 February	Complete any tables and graphs and write the discussion
13 February	Complete the report leaving time to proofread and edit the work
14 February	Submit

colour coding as you feel necessary, perhaps even showing day-by-day activities rather than a weekly plan, if this helps you.

From your term planner you should be able to see all your submission dates. It's good to have a list of when all your assignments are due so you can work to those deadlines. But then try and break those deadlines down into smaller achievable goals. For example, you have two weeks to complete a report on 'Measuring energy expenditure' that is due to be submitted on 16 February, so you could break this down into more workable chunks as shown in Table 8.2.

You could do this for all your assignments or just the larger ones. Having small realistic targets means can you achieve them, tick them off and then build on them towards your larger goal; with every achievement you will probably find that your confidence grows too.

We have also learnt that you need to use time when you have it. It is tempting to leave work until you have a clear day or an afternoon, but actually if you have a spare 30 minutes here and there you will be surprised how much you can get done.

Files

We know we don't have to tell you about how important it is to save your work. But do take some time to think about where you are saving the work and how you can ensure you can find it again easily.

If you are working in a university computer suite, are you trying to save your work to the computer you are working on or are you saving it to a place on the university network? Just double checking, using the 'save as' function, can save you problems and heartache later.

It's also worth having a USB stick, flash drive or a portable hard drive where you can save work, particularly if you are likely to have to move computers regularly; but take care of your USB stick, as they are easy to lose, and make sure it is password protected too. You might also consider cloud-based storage options. Another 'hack' we recommend is emailing your work to yourself so you can access it that way and have a backup.

Name new files with something you will identify next time, not just with your name. In fact, most work now has to be submitted anonymously so it is probably better if your name is not included in the file. But do make sure the file name is recognisable and will make sense to you if you had to come back to it in a month's time or when you want to start revising.

Just as you would have separate binders or card dividers for all your paper notes and handouts, use folders in your computer's file manager directory to organise your electronic files. Perhaps a new folder for each module you are studying will help keep your files organised and easy to locate and manage.

If there are websites you regularly return to, use the 'history' function or create bookmarks; this is convenient but also saves time. If you have a lot of bookmarks you might want to organise them into folders.

Take a look at how many tabs you have open on your browser. If you are someone who opens lots of tabs, try to remember to close them when you have finished as this will make things easier to find and also save time at the end of your study session.

If you are making notes and you want to link to a certain webpage, or to a different place in your document, you can always use a hyperlink. In MS Word look for the hyperlink icon in the tool bar under the 'insert' tab.

For keeping your references organised, you might want to use some sort of reference manager such Refworks™, Endnote™ or Mendeley™, for example. They can help keep a track of all the journal papers you have accumulated and will also help you when it comes to writing your reference list or bibliography.

Finally, it goes without saying, always make sure your computer or laptop is password protected.

Virtual learning environments

It is most likely that the university you are studying at will use some form of virtual learning environment (VLE) for online teaching. Different VLE platforms include Blackboard, Brightspace, Moodle, MS teams. Different universities may use different platforms or may even use a combination. It is a good use of time to get familiar with the ones you will be using before the lecture, as this is where most of the materials you will need will be placed. Make sure you can navigate around the VLE so you can find all the relevant materials you will need for your course.

VLEs usually host all the teaching materials, which might include:

* Module or course handbook
* Lecture notes

- Links or access points for live lectures
- Reading and resource lists
- Journal papers
- Quizzes
- Past exam papers
- Other activities
- An announcement or chat area
- The VLE might also host the submission box where you upload and submit assessments

Check the VLE regularly as you might find useful documents suddenly appear and it is a good idea to check the announcements to make sure you don't miss anything.

The VLE may also be the place where you can interact and communicate with your lecturers and fellow students. This might be in lectures, seminars or even collaborating on a group project or on message boards.

Online lectures

If it's a live teaching activity, a camera and a microphone will be very useful for interacting. It is usually good to start off with your microphone muted, as background noise can affect a lecture or meeting. Usually, the lecturer will invite you to turn on your microphone at an appropriate time so you can contribute to any discussions and ask questions. Most platforms have an icon where you can wave your hand to indicate you have a query or a chat function where you can type in your questions.

We know it is not always possible for you to turn your camera on. Not all laptops have built in-cameras, or you just may not be comfortable with it. Your lecturers should be understanding about this issue. However, lecturers do like being able to see their students where possible so we can see if you are enjoying the lecture or perhaps are confused and need further clarification.

But do make sure you are prepared and dressed appropriately. No matter how tempting it may be to watch a lecture in bed in your pyjamas, get up and get dressed. You will feel that you are in work mode and will then act like you are in work mode, be more motivated and will absorb and learn more from the class.

Active learning

Keep your learning active. Active learning can help ensure you stay engaged and improve your knowledge retention (Michael 2006). Active learning might include ensuring you do your reading, problem-solving activities or answering questions, even taking lecture notes and summarising information can be active.

It is easy to think you can watch a lecture like you would a television programme, especially since in many cases you can go back to the recordings later. However, this is not necessarily the best way to engage with material and really learn it. Just as you would in an on-campus lecture, making notes using pen and paper can help with focus, as it forces you to summarise what you are listening to in your own words. Furthermore, the act of writing is associated with greater cognitive understanding and better recall according to van der Velden (2021).

Some students struggle to read on screen, so if you are someone who prefers to read on paper then you can always print your papers out for reading or adding notes to. There are also 'text to speech' packages such as Claro Software™ that will read online print out loud.

Online tutorials

Online tutorials are an opportunity to talk to your lecturer/tutor and/or other students. Although using your camera during a tutorial can be friendlier and make discussions easier, we know it is not always easy or appropriate to use the camera. However, you can ensure you display your name and, in many cases, show a profile picture. Ideally try to attend all tutorials if you can. This way you can ask questions and get involved; however, if this is difficult it may be possible to view a recording later.

At the end of the tutorial make sure you close the programmes carefully; sometimes there is more than one tab to close to ensure you are fully logged out.

Breakout rooms

Some lecturers may arrange online breakout rooms to divide the class into smaller groups for seminar-style discussions or to work on a particular task. A breakout room is usually separate from the main online lecture room. Only those in a particular breakout room can hear the discussion, so it is slightly more private. However, in some VLEs it is possible to move between breakout rooms if the lecturer allows this, and usually the lecturer can pop into all the breakout rooms or send messages into the rooms too. Don't just leave the session when the lecturer divides the class into breakout rooms. This is a good opportunity for networking, to meet and chat with other students, talk about your studies and offer peer-to-peer support. Your participation is important and highlights your ability to work as part of a team with a common purpose.

Discussion and study groups

At times, online study might make you feel a bit isolated, but it does not have to be like that, so do look for opportunities to engage with other students on the course. You should attend the live lectures and seminars where it will be possible to video chat with others, including the lecturer. Do also try to actively participate in any online discussion groups; this could be in a chat or posting a question on a discussion board. Discussion boards allow you to interact asynchronously, even outside of usual class times, and offer another opportunity to engage with the topic. New threads may be created for different topics. Because you can post a message any time, you have more time to think about what you want to post and discussions can be less formal than in a scheduled class. Remember to keep your messages clear and concise and be respectful of the opinions of others. Try not to interact with the same few classmates, but debate with others in the same class to get diverse opinions (Roper 2007). Avoid posts such as 'good point' or just 'I agree'; try to add something to the discussion if you can. Getting involved in relevant and topical discussions can also help you feel involved and motivated.

Just as you can organise your own study groups when physically in the university, there is no reason why you cannot set up your own online study group using Zoom or Skype, for example. You could build a supportive student network, or revision group or a reading circle. These can be both motivational and supportive too.

Although many universities do not support WhatsApp, it is a method that students often use to chat more informally. Treat this as you would the more formal methods of communication; think before you send a message and always be respectful and kind.

Online assessments

Many of your assessments will be online. This could be an online multiple-choice test or an exam, but equally it could be an essay or any other type of assessment.

Most universities have a software system such as Turnitin™ where you upload your work for marking. Not only is this where you will get your marks and feedback, but it also runs a plagiarism check on your work against other work that has been submitted at your university and other institutions as well as online materials.

Make sure you know where to access the submission or test points well in advance of your assessment deadline. In most cases it will be on the VLE platform you are familiar with, but double check to be on the safe side.

Other online services

There may be other online resources you will need to access frequently. This may include the university website. There is usually a student portal or an area where current students can log in and find out information about services including the students' union, wellbeing support, finance, registry, etc.

The other online place you will probably need to use heavily is the library. Here you can search the catalogues, access e-books and also journal collections, including e-journals. There is likely to be a virtual librarian or someone you can email if you have any questions or need advice.

Emails

When not in class, your university will probably communicate with you through email. In most cases they will use your university email address and not a personal email address, so do make sure you check your university account regularly.

Be professional and keep your emails relatively formal. For example, start an email with 'Dear Dr ...' and not 'Hi' and definitely do not use 'Hey' to start an email to your lecturer. At least to begin with, ensure you provide adequate information including your name, programme, year group and the module you are referring to. We have lost count of how many emails we get saying 'in the nutrition module'; between us we teach about 10 different nutrition modules, so be sure to state which one you mean.

Ideally, write grammatically correct sentences out in full, rather than using abbreviations the way you might write a text; an occasional emoji might provide some light relief but don't overdo it. Avoid writing in capitals.

Give your email an appropriate and meaningful subject heading and try to keep the body of your email concise and to the point.

Think before you send. If we are not 100 per cent sure about an email we sometimes email them to ourselves, then sleep on it and review the email the next day before deciding to send to the intended recipient. Always consider how the content of the email would be received if you were to say the same thing face to face.

When replying to emails, check if are you replying just to the sender or if you are replying to all on the email list. If you only need to respond to one or two of the names listed then just do that; don't fill up everyone else's email box. Also check that 'Reply all' is not set as a default in your settings.

Do you know the difference between CC and BCC? CC stands for carbon copy (from the days of using typewriters with carbon paper to make a carbon copy), and this is often used when you are copying someone in for information purposes. BCC (blind carbon copy) can be used to hide who else is in the message; this could be used when you don't want to share email addresses and want to keep those addresses private. Although if you do need to email large groups, or use addresses from a mailing list, you can usually set up a mail merge that also can be personalised.

Try to keep your email account tidy, delete unnecessary emails and put those you want to keep in appropriately named folders; otherwise the volume of emails can become overwhelming.

It is tempting to have email notifications permanently switched on, but would you be more productive if you restricted email checking to certain times, say once or twice a day?

Although many staff do often work late and at weekends you should not expect a reply to an email at those times. Ideally send your email during core working hours, although we realise that you may need to work flexibly too. So, if you cannot put a delay on the email, then send it but do not expect an immediate response and allow a reasonable amount of time for an email reply. Anecdotally, staff report receiving up to 100 emails a day; so ask yourself if you need to send that email and also understand that a reply may take a little time.

Online conferences and webinars

As result of the COVID-19 pandemic, many conferences were forced to move online and many have continued to provide this option. This was a great opportunity for students to attend conferences, hear about up-to-date research and network with others in the field, without the additional cost of travel. Check the Association for Nutrition and British Dietetic Associations' webpages to see if there are any relevant conferences coming up.

There has also been an increase in the number of online webinars given by experts. These are another way to increase your knowledge of particular topics and keep your continuing professional development (CPD) up to date from the comfort of your own home.

Staying safe online

There are certain things you should always do to stay safe in the online world.

Make your passwords difficult to hack, using a combination of letters, numbers and character keys. Always change any default passwords and change your password immediately if you think your account may have been accessed or compromised. Never give password details, or your PIN, to anyone and do not allow your browser to store passwords either. Check your privacy settings on all your devices as well as your location services or any geo-locator settings too.

Keep your software and antivirus protection up to date and recognise the risks of using unsecured public Wi-Fi connections. Be aware of potential phishing scams; never click on an emailed link unless you are completely sure of the sender.

Think before you post anything online. Block unsuitable content and set filters on your home Wi-Fi. If you have experienced or witnessed any form of cyberbullying, you should take screenshots as evidence and report this to the platform. The Citizens Advice Bureau and the police can also provide further guidance on online harassment.

If you would like further information, see the UK government website on how you can protect yourself from fraud and cyber-crime (Home Office 2020).

Your wellbeing

If you need help with online study, there is always someone you can ask. First there is your tutor, or perhaps the course leader. The university may also have people who can help with specific applications, e-learning in general or library services. Early on in your studies you should find out who these people are and how to contact them.

As with any type of study, ensure you take regular breaks. You may want to take a break from all electronic devices from time to time as well, so turn off notifications or activate your 'do not disturb' notice. It is important to stay hydrated and eat well whilst you are studying, so do this away from your computer. You should also try to do some form of physical activity and get some fresh air, if possible, too.

Summary

Hopefully this chapter has given you suggestions for everything you need to study online successfully. Think about where you are going to work, plan your time, and organise your files and documents. You may also now know a bit more about VLEs and how online lectures and tutorials can work. Also, consider how you interact and communicate online and stay safe and well.

Reflective questions

- Do you have a system for saving your work and files safely?
- Do you know which VLE your university uses and are you familiar with it?
- Are you staying safe online?

Suggested further reading

Home Office (2020) Fraud and cybercrime. Available at: https://www.gov.uk/government/publications/coronavirus-covid-19-fraud-and-cyber-crime
Open University (2020) Study skills for online learning. Available at: https://help.open.ac.uk/browse/computing/study-skills-for-online-learning

References

Home Office (2020) Fraud and cybercrime. Available at: https://www.gov.uk/government/publications/coronavirus-covid-19-fraud-and-cyber-crime (accessed 15 March 2021).

Michael, J. (2006) Where's the evidence that active learning works? *Advances in Physiology Education*, 30: 159–67.

Roper, A. (2007) How students develop online learning skills, *Educause Quarterly*, 1: 62–65.

van der Velden, M. (2021) 'I felt a new connection between my fingers and brain': a thematic analysis of student reflections on the use of pen and paper during lectures, *Teaching in Higher Education*. doi: 10.1080/13562517.2020.1863347 (accessed 4 November 2021).

9 Feedback and reflection

Overview and outline

This chapter will explain what feedback is and the different types of feedback you may experience. It is important to reflect on feedback, so we will outline different ways of doing this by drawing upon popular reflective models including those created by the academics Schön, Gibbs and Kolb that can be used to reflect on the learning process. You may want to create a feedback portfolio so you can monitor your progress. Hopefully this will help you further develop your own reflective skills, so you are able to use feedback constructively and even provide your own feedback to improve your future assessments and work.

What is feedback?

Many students think that feedback is the grade or comments you receive on a piece of work you have submitted for marking. This is correct but feedback can take many other forms. Feedback can be written; it can be verbal; it might be given in class or online. Even a chat in the corridor with a lecturer or another student could provide you with essential feedback that should not be ignored.

The feedback you receive may include:

- A mark or grade
- Comments written on an assessment online
- Comments written on paper
- A marking template
- A marking matrix
- A cover sheet
- Oral feedback
- Audio feedback
- Discussion in a small group, e.g. a tutorial or a seminar
- Email from a lecturer
- Informal chat with a lecturer

- Discussions with peers
- Written comments from other students (peer assessment)
- The critique you give yourself when comparing your work to your peers, the marking criteria or an exemplar

All these different types of feedback, whether the feedback is positive or negative, can provide you with the information and encouragement you need to do even better.

Feedback has been described as a process where the student makes sense of performance information to further their learning (Henderson et al. 2019). This definition emphasises the fact that feedback is an important part of learning. It is not just about pointing out errors; it should be a guide to help you make sense of your learning and ideally encourage reflective practice (more about this later). Although it is easy to think that feedback is simply information from a lecturer about your assessment, it can be much more of a long-term dialogue (Price et al. 2011) that is part of your whole learning experience.

Formative and summative feedback

You may have come across formative and summative assessment. Formative assessments are usually the smaller pieces of work you do as you are going along to monitor your understanding. Summative assessments, on the other hand, evaluate what you have learnt and are often at the end of the course. Well, there is also formative and summative feedback (Race 2007). You may pick up formative feedback throughout your course and this might include in-class discussions, tutorials, conversations or emails from lecturers or other students, or even written comments on drafts. Summative feedback is usually the final grade or feedback on a piece of work you have submitted or an exam you have taken. Look out for, and be open to, formative feedback throughout your course; it will help you with the summative assessments and build your confidence, but it can also help you make sense of the summative feedback you get at a later date.

Don't just look at the mark!

When you get your work back it is very easy to become focused on the mark; but don't just check your percentage score, take a detailed look at the feedback you have been given. In fact, the comments are arguably much more important than the grade or mark. Your lecturers probably spent a lot of time providing individual feedback to help explain your mark and show you how to improve on your next piece of work. Lecturers and supervisors want to help you improve and often spend hours editing and commenting on a piece of work, so please try to take those comments on board to avoid making the very same mistakes on your next assessment. Read and consider the comments. Re-read the comments and think about what they mean then decide what you need to keep doing and what you need to change or develop in order to move forward.

For example, if referencing is frequently mentioned: could you find a copy of your university's referencing guide and go through it; could you attend a workshop on referencing; or could you ask your tutor for advice?

Even if you did really well, you can still learn from the feedback, to work out what it was that got you that top mark, how to maintain that high standard and possibly do even better next time.

With the advent of online learning and assessment, we can usually see when a student has accessed their feedback and a surprising number do not even open the file to look at the feedback and comments provided by the lecturer. They are therefore missing out on crucial information that could instantly help them improve their marks on future assessments.

Take a step back

It has been shown that attitude to feedback and the person who gave you that feedback can influence academic performance (Forsythe and Johnson 2017), and as such this can motivate or demotivate you; so use that knowledge to consider how that feedback can be used and make sure it inspires you to do even better.

When you first get your feedback, it may occasionally be a surprise or even cause you to be upset and, if this is the case, put the work away and come back to it later or another day. However, don't leave it too long or you will be absorbed in your next assessment, forget to go back and could end up making the same mistakes again.

It might comfort you to know that your lecturers may have the same reaction when they submit a paper to a journal and then get back the reviewers' comments. 'Reviewer 2' is a meme and infamous in academia and on social media for providing harsh or irrelevant comments. But in these cases, and when it has happened to us, we usually find if we put the review aside and then pick it up again the next day with fresh eyes, those comments weren't nearly as bad as first thought.

Try not to over-analyse remarks made in relation to assessments you know you have worked hard on; take them at face value. It is very easy to over interpret what they mean or take them personally. But in most cases the work would have been marked anonymously and, although on occasion comments may be badly written or seem blunt, they are designed to be constructive and not an attack. Look for the positive comments and not just the negative ones; it's very easy to focus on minor mistakes and not congratulate yourself on what you did well. You want to ensure you continue doing the things you got right in addition to what you might do differently. It is worth making a note of any constructive annotations and useful observations. Finally (irrespective of how much effort you think you put in) ask yourself, is the mark given justified?

Activity

How can you improve your next piece of work?

Reflect on a recent piece of assessment that was given feedback and ask yourself the following questions:

- What went well?
- What would you do differently?
- How will this change what you do in the future?
- Has your opinion or outlook changed?

Feedback can be bi-directional and collaborative, perhaps part of a wider conversation. A good example of this would be a conversation with your peers. You might even share your feedback with other students. You can learn from each other's mistakes but also help each other understand what the comments mean; not everyone will feel comfortable doing this, so do respect each other's need for privacy if required. You can also chat to your tutor about your feedback too. If you don't understand a comment, then it is perfectly acceptable to contact the marker to discuss it and get clarification. Perhaps they have not explained themselves as well as they could have, and often a quick conversation could clear up any concerns on both sides. In fact, you do not have to wait until feedback is given – you are perfectly entitled to ask for feedback.

Using the marking criteria before and after submitting a piece of work

The person marking your work is probably using a marking criteria (or a marking scheme) to ensure that their marking decisions are consistent with predetermined standards. Lecturers do this to make sure the marking is transparent and fair. You should take some time to look at the marking criteria carefully and use it to ensure you know what is expected of you; but also it can help you look at your work in a way similar to the person marking it.

Obviously, you want to use the marking criteria when you are completing your work, to ensure you are doing what is asked, but it can be worth going back to that marking criteria after you have received feedback to see how your work compares. You can also use the criteria to help you identify what you need to do differently, or more of, in order to move up to the next grade boundary. You can even use the marking criteria to mark your own work and start to develop your own feedback skills.

Develop your own feedback skills

Once you get familiar with reviewing your marked work, understanding the comments and acting on feedback, you can start to think about how you might develop your own personal feedback skills. This can be a very useful skill, as after you graduate you will have to keep your knowledge and skills up to date with continuing professional development (CPD). You will need to provide your own feedback on what you learnt and what you could do differently (also see Chapter 14 on CPD).

Reflection

Reflection is essentially thinking about a certain event or piece of work, making sense of it, learning from experience, then using that to create actions or ideas as to what you could do differently next time to get an even better outcome. It can be an important part of the learning process and a key skill you can use not only at university but also throughout your career.

John Dewey was an educational psychologist and philosopher who was one of the first to consider reflection in relation to learning. He thought that reflection could help students make sense of things they found confusing; essentially it could enable students to move from a state of perplexity to equilibrium (Dewey 1933). He also thought reflection was something that could be practised and perfected, so it is something that will get easier the more often you do it.

Building on the foundations of Dewey's work, there are many models of reflection you can use to help you consider your strengths and weaknesses and set appropriate targets. In doing so you can use and create your own feedback in a structured way. Some of the most well-known of these models of reflection are outlined below.

Gibb's reflective cycle

Back in the 1980s a university lecturer called Graham Gibbs put forward the 'Reflective Cycle' (Gibbs 1988). This cycle can be considered a framework for examining repeated experiences. There are six key stages as shown in Fig. 9.1.

The six key stages can be described as follows:

1 **Description** – of the experience, event or piece of work
2 **Feelings** – your thoughts and feelings on that experience
3 **Evaluation** – of that experience, this should include good and bad
4 **Analysis** – how you can make sense of the situation
5 **Conclusion** – what you learnt and what you could have done differently
6 **Action plan** – how you would deal with a similar situation in the future or any general changes that would be appropriate.

Figure 9.1 Gibbs' cycle of reflection (Gibbs 1988)

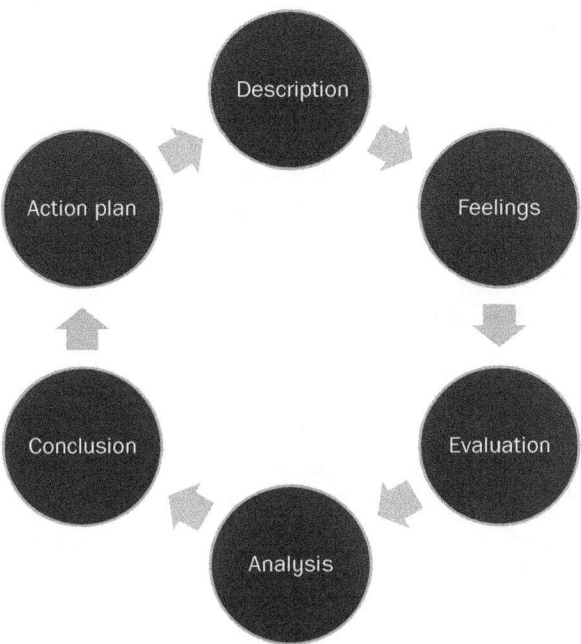

Gibbs' reflective cycle can be a very useful guide as to the thought process, particularly if you are not used to reflective practice. It can be applied to situations that you know will come up again and where you want to improve. Many lecturers use this cycle to reflect on how a teaching session may have gone, to improve their lecturing skills, but it can be very useful for students too. It can be applied to a piece of work or a presentation, for example, which you want to learn from and get better at. As with everything it can take practice, but the more you use this reflective cycle the easier it will become.

Schön's theory

If you prefer a simpler model, then Schön's (1983) theory is arguably less open to misinterpretation. It could be described as a linear framework for thinking and less of a step-by-step process than some of the other models. But some students may find it useful for helping to put their thoughts in order. The idea here is that there are basically two types of reflection: 'reflection in action' and 'reflection on action'.

Essentially, there is the reflection that happens during an event and the reflection that happens after an event.

So, think about what you feel while you are doing something, e.g. perhaps whilst in a lecture or during a presentation. Later think about what happened, what else do you know that might help and what would you do differently next time?

Table 9.1   Reflection in action and reflection on action

Reflection in action (at the time)	Reflection on action (after)
The experience	Thinking and reviewing what has happened
Thinking at the time	What would you do differently next time
Deciding how to act at the time	Incorporating new information
Acting instantly	Using new ideas to inform the experience

Look at the two boxed examples.

During the event (reflection in action)

You are in an exam, you are running out of time and notice you only have 5 minutes left to complete your essay on 'glycolysis'.

- You know you haven't got time to write everything out in full so you make bullet points of the key things you want to mention
- You think a diagram would be a quicker way of showing how ATP is generated, so you draw this.

After the event (reflection on action)

You consider what happened during the exam and what you could do differently next time.

- You didn't keep an eye on the clock so next time you will work out how long you have for each question and stick to this.
- Your hand got tired and your writing became slower; you could practise writing revision notes by hand so you are used to it.
- You didn't know all the details of glycolysis as well as you could have, so you waffled which took longer, you could look again at your revision strategy.
- However, you did include a diagram, which you think helped illustrate some points well.

Kolb's learning cycle

If you prefer slightly more guidance you may prefer Kolb's learning cycle. This is widely recognised and based on the concept of 'Experiential Learning Theory' (Kolb and Kolb 2018); as such it is based on the idea that you need experience to learn.

Figure 9.2 Kolb's learning cycle (adapted from Kolb 1984; Kolb and Kolb 2018)

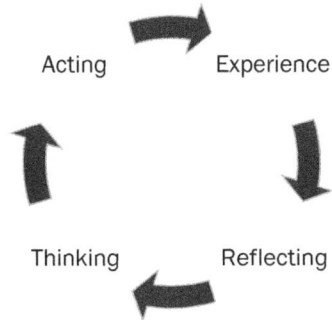

Acting Experience

Thinking Reflecting

There are four key points:

1 **Experience** – *this is the actual doing* – for example writing an essay, doing an exam or a presentation.
2 **Reflecting** – *observations and reflections* – what you noticed that you did, for example you got your referencing wrong, ran out of time, or read from notes not looking up.
3 **Thinking** – *the development of ideas* – this is where you learn from experience, for example from feedback or talking to your peers and your tutor.
4 **Acting** – *testing ideas in practice* – trialling what you have since learnt, such as learning how to reference correctly, set time limits for each question, practising your presentation so you can remember more and look up.

In theory you could start at any of the points in the cycle but usually it starts with 'Experience'. The concept is that the learning cycle is ongoing and not a linear process; in fact, you could even be at more than one of the points at any given time.

There are many adaptations of these models and you may have come across other models during your studies. The most important thing is to think about which one suits you best and would be the easiest for you to put into action, therefore allowing you to get the most from it.

Feedback portfolio

Some lecturers recommend that students create and collate a feedback portfolio (Winstone and Boud 2020). This is one way of tracking your learning journey. It could help you monitor your progress, encourage reflection and also identify what you can do to improve your next pieces of work. A portfolio can help you recognise your personal development and, help you recognise changes in other outcomes such as self-confidence and employability

(Winstone 2019). You can include any type of feedback; it doesn't just have to be that from assessed work. You can even include marking criteria, so you know how work has been assessed. The portfolio could be online or print, whatever suits you best, but ideally it should be easily accessed so you can add to it regularly over time.

Portfolios can be particularly useful for collating feedback when you have a modular programme or degree, to ensure you apply your learning from previous modules to the modules you are currently studying. Portfolios also encourage feedforward, i.e. constructive ideas and suggestions that can be used to benefit your work before you submit it. By reflecting on your previous feedback on all modules you can identify themes and use this to improve future work.

You can even combine your feedback portfolio with your record of CPD, as both require you to reflect on what you have learnt and what you will take forward with you (see Chapter 14).

Summary

Formative and summative feedback can be given in many different forms; it is more than just a grade or written comments on an essay. Feedback can help inform your learning experience and inspire you to achieve more. Reflecting on your feedback can help to identify what you need to do next and several models of reflection were outlined to help you find the one that suits you best.

Reflective questions

- Have you considered the different types of feedback you have received?
- Could you go back and look at your feedback on different pieces of assessment – were there any common themes or comments?
- Which model of reflection did you find easiest to follow and that best suits your personal learning style? Could you apply to it an assessment you found challenging?

Suggested further reading

Hepplestone, S., Parkin, H., Irwin, B. et al. (2010) *A Student Guide to Using Feedback*. Sheffield: Learning and Teaching Institute, Sheffield Hallam University. Available at: https://evidencenet.pbworks.com/f/guide+for+students+FINAL.pdf (accessed 15 January 2021).

References

Dewey, J. (1933) *How We Think: A Restatement of the Relation of Reflective Thinking to the Educative Process*. Boston: D.C. Heath and Company.

Forsythe, A. and Johnson, S. (2017) Thanks, but no-thanks for the feedback, *Assessment & Evaluation in Higher Education*, 42(6): 850–59. doi: 10.1080/02602938.2016.1202190 (accessed 5 November 2021).

Gibbs, G. (1988). *Learning by Doing: A Guide to Teaching and Learning Methods*. London: Further Education Unit.

Henderson, M., Molloy, E., Ajjawi, R. and Boud, D. (2019) Designing feedback for impact, in M. Henderson, R. Ajjawi, D. Boud and E. Mollo (eds) *The Impact of Feedback in Higher Education*. London: Palgrave Macmillan.

Kolb, D.A. (1984) *Experiential Learning: Experience as the source of learning and development*. Englewood Cliffs, NJ: Prentice Hall.

Kolb, A. and Kolb, D. (2018) Eight important things to know about the experiential learning cycle, *Australian Educational Leader*, 40(3). Available at: https://learningfromexperience.com/downloads/research-library/eight-important-things-to-know-about-the-experiential-learning-cycle.pdf (accessed 7 January 2021).

Price, M., Handley, K. and Millar, J. (2011) Feedback: focusing attention on engagement, *Studies in Higher Education*, 36(8): 879–96. doi: 10.1080/03075079.2010.483513 (accessed 05 November 2021).

Race, P. (2007) *How to Get a Good Degree*, 2nd edn. Maidenhead: Open University Press.

Schön, D. A. (1983) *The Reflective Practitioner: How Professionals Think in Action*. New York: Basic Books. (Reprinted in 1995.)

Winstone, N.E. (2019) Facilitating students' use of feedback: capturing and tracking impact using digital tools, in M. Henderson, R. Ajjawi, D. Boud and E. Mollo (eds) *The Impact of Feedback in Higher Education*. London: Palgrave.

Winstone, N.E. and Boud, D. (2020) The need to disentangle assessment and feedback in higher education, *Studies in Higher Education*. doi: 10.1080/03075079.2020.1779687.

Part B

10 Being a graduate

Overview and outline

Being a graduate provides you with an academic qualification but, in addition to your degree, you will also have acquired other valuable skills. This chapter asks you to consider what transferable skills you have gained alongside work and volunteering experience and how to highlight these qualities when applying for jobs and/or postgraduate study. You will want a strong *curriculum vitae* (CV) and personal statement but you also need to think about where jobs will be advertised. Moreover, this chapter will ask you to think about how you present yourself to the world on different social media platforms, whilst ensuring your posts are evidence based and professional.

Being a graduate?

Being a graduate can be a confusing time. You may be celebrating the completion of your degree, but you may also be sad to be leaving university and simultaneously excited or nervous about what the future may bring. But being a graduate isn't just about your academic qualification: it also reflects the qualities that a graduate would be expected to have, such as the specific skills and abilities that you developed throughout your time at university and which have developed with experience. These are the skills and qualities that will make you employable.

It is never too early to think about what you would like to do when you graduate. With some foresight and planning whilst you are studying for your degree, you can make your chosen path clearer and enhance your chances of achieving your career aspirations.

Consider your options

Many of you may already know that you want to become a Dietitian or a Registered Nutritionist; you probably chose your degree programme to reflect this. But even within the fields of nutrition and dietetics there are a variety of different pathways.

Career possibilities in nutrition and dietetics include:

- Academia
- Animal nutrition
- Catering
- Community Dietitian or Nutritionist
- Dietitian – various specialities
- Food technologist
- Health Promotion Officer
- International nutrition
- Nutrition research
- Nutritionist in industry
- Public Health Nutritionist
- Sports and exercise nutrition

Furthermore, your ideas may change over the course of your degree and there is certainly no harm in exploring all your options. Perhaps you want to consider other careers, such as the civil service, teaching or graduate training schemes, etc. Think broadly at this stage, consider applying for different opportunities that come your way and are of interest.

The next thing to think about is where vacancies are likely to be advertised, so you can see the different types of jobs that exist. Think about searching professional association websites, newspapers, scientific and industry magazines, recruitment agencies, employer's websites; for example, for jobs in hospitals try the NHS website: https://www.jobs.nhs.uk/. Visit your university careers centre, which often lists current vacancies and can offer ideas for where to target your search. You should also ensure you attend your university careers fairs, where there will usually be a range of employers that you can chat to about different roles and get their advice on what they look for in potential employees.

Alternatively, perhaps you want to do a postgraduate degree such as a master's degree or a PhD before you start work in the field.

Postgraduate study

Considering whether to do postgraduate study can be a big decision, not least because of the time and the financial investments involved. So ensure you have a clear reason for wanting to study further. Will having a postgraduate qualification make it easier to get into your dream career or are you just not sure you are ready to move full time into the world of work?

There are many different types of postgraduate courses:

- **Postgraduate diplomas** (PGDip) are usually the same level as a master's degree but shorter (two-thirds as long). It is possible to get into Dietetics with a postgraduate diploma at certain universities or you can do a master's course.

- **Master's** courses can further your knowledge in an area related to your degree or they can be conversion courses and introduce you to a new area of study, e.g. computing or law. Most MSc masters are usually taught with lectures, seminars and a dissertation, but there are other types now available such as an MRes where a greater emphasis is given to research. An MPhil is usually pure research and may be a stepping stone to a PhD. So think carefully about which type of master's course would be best for you.

- **PhD**: some universities will allow you to go straight from your undergraduate degree onto a PhD but other universities prefer you to have gained a master's degree first.

Check the entry requirements for any course you are interested in. Most will expect a least a 2: ii grade in your undergraduate degree and, depending on the popularity of particular courses and place limitations, the qualification criteria may be higher.

Same or different university? There are many advantages to staying to do a postgraduate course at the same university where you did your undergraduate course: you will know your way around, you will have the same email and learning platforms, and you will probably know the staff too. However, moving to another university will mean you can broaden your network and get to know more students and staff; they may also have different specialisms and so it is worth investigating this.

Once you have decided what you want to do next you can think about presenting yourself in the best light in the applications and highlighting your qualifications and skills. But first you need to recognise the many skills you have developed.

Recognising your skills

Soft skills are those transferable skills that you acquire alongside your degree, such as presentation or organisational skills, but equally can be skills that you developed as part of your Saturday job or through volunteering etc. Although not a qualification in themselves they can be highly regarded by employers. Many of these skills have already been outlined in this book; they may also have been specified in the module descriptions of the courses you are currently studying. Soft skills can cover many areas and may include:

- Adaptability
- Analytical skills
- Commercial awareness
- Communication
- Decision making
- Flexibility

- Initiative
- Innovation
- IT skills
- Leadership
- Negotiation
- Networking
- Numeracy skills
- Organisation
- Presentation
- Problem solving
- Research
- Teamwork
- Time management

(List based on information from the University of Manchester Careers Service 2021).

You will develop these soft skills as you progress through your studies, as you have different experiences, and from advice or increased awareness of different opinions (Neves 2018), but do keep a track of the skills you have developed and achieved.

Complete a skills audit

A skills audit can help you identify and evaluate the skills you already have and those you would like to develop and progress. Table 10.1 shows an example of what a skills audit could look like.

As you recognise and develop these skills you may want to consider how best you can include and highlight them on any job application forms or your CV.

Table 10.1   Example of a skills audit

Skill	Evidence	Score (1–4)*	Progress
Teamwork	Led group project that was given an A grade	2	Confident enough to be team leader
Time management	Handing in coursework on time	1	All work to date submitted on time

*Where 1 = lots of experience, 2 = some experience, 3 = little experience, 4 = no experience

CV

You should make the most of your university careers centre. The staff will be delighted to help you put together a CV; they may even have an electronic CV builder. They can also give you lots of tips for ensuring it is well presented and contains all the required key information. But some general pointers are provided here.

Your CV should include the following details:

Personal details: put your name in a bigger font than the other information so that it stands out. Include your contact details, but it is usually recommended that you avoid including your age or gender as neither affects your ability to do the job.

Personal profile: this should state who you are, your skills and your aims. Keep this concise – around four sentences long.

Education: give this in reverse chronological order, so your most recent achievement is seen first. Include details of qualification, subject, grade, place of study with dates. Also include any other types of training here too.

Work experience: put the job title, the company and the dates in bold. Underneath, briefly describe your key duties; provide more details for very relevant experience, less information for less important experience.

Key achievements: this can include special awards, such as graduate or dissertation prizes, publications or any examples of where you have had a positive impact – don't be modest. This can be a separate section or you could include this information under the appropriate qualification or particular jobs.

Key skills: you should put here skills such as languages, first aid, IT and also your employability skills. Where possible, match your skills to the role for which you are applying and try to show evidence for the skills you have listed.

Interests: you want to show that you have a well-rounded personality but keep this section brief and include nothing that could be considered controversial.

References: give the name and brief contact details; this is far better than 'on request'. But do ask permission first from people if you want them to be referees for you.

Remember to ensure your CV is presented in a straightforward manner with clear headings. It is likely to be skim read initially; it is possible that a machine will read it before a person does, so you need it to be clear and well laid out. Check your spelling and grammar and then get someone else to check it for you. Remember that your CV will be used to judge your writing skills as well as your presentation skills. Try to keep it to two pages unless you are going for a more senior position which might require more information.

You should adapt your CV for specific job opportunities, highlighting the points most relevant to the job you are applying for. Remember it is your CV that will get you to the interview stage of any job application.

Application forms

Many job adverts will ask you to complete an application form as well as or instead of a CV.

If you have your CV ready you may be able to copy and paste some of that information straight into an application form; but be careful to ensure you have read the question carefully so that the pasted information fits appropriately and is strictly relevant. Take your time to read and complete the form carefully.

The application form may ask for a personal statement. Often you have had to put so much information into an application form, under different sections, such as qualifications and work experience, that by the time you get to the personal statement it is easy to think you have already included all the relevant information you need. However, the employer will probably give this section the most attention, so it is really important to reiterate key information here and in particular make your statement relevant to the job description. As with your CV, double check your spelling and grammar.

Work experience

Think about your experience in broad terms. One of our students told us she had only ever worked in a supermarket and did not think this was worth putting on her CV. But consider the skills that such a job includes: customer service, communication, product knowledge, being a team player, financial responsibilities, trustworthiness, time management, possibly even leadership. Any work experience is good experience and you should make sure you include it on your CV. It can be tricky finding work experience, but experience can be gained in many different ways; for example do you have a part-time job, do you have a role in a university society, tutoring fellow students, are you the course rep or could you volunteer?

Volunteering

Volunteering can help you gain relevant experience, provide life skills and really make a difference. It can make you look proactive and enthusiastic, qualities that many employers will be looking for and hence can be a great thing to add to your CV. It can also be a good way to network and meet people. Perhaps your university has a volunteering scheme, but you could also consider local hospitals, charities, nursing homes, schools and community kitchens and groups. Many food banks are unfortunately desperate for volunteers and all these places mentioned could provide relevant experience for anyone wanting to work in nutrition and dietetics. As if you needed any more reasons to get involved, students who volunteer whilst at university have stated that they gained satisfaction from helping others, reported improved mental wellbeing and were more likely to meet physical activity guidelines (Bhardwa 2018; Lederer et al. 2015).

Networking

As you consider your future career, think about what contacts you have and what contacts your university may have. Many universities organise careers fairs where they invite a variety of employers to visit the university, or they may have information about regional careers fairs that you could attend. Also make use of your university's alumni; some careers centres even have mentoring schemes where they can pair you up with someone working in the field that you are interested in.

Look out for any relevant conferences. Conferences can be a great way to learn more about your field but also an opportunity to speak with people working in that field and ask questions. There are usually coffee breaks and sometimes social activities that are designed to provide opportunities to meet other people.

Using social media

Social media consists of interactive computer-based technologies and platforms that allow sharing of information within online communities and networks. It can provide another way of networking, for example through LinkedIn.

LinkedIn

LinkedIn is a type of social network for different professionals to connect and share. It is a way of networking online that enables individuals to connect with each other in a professional setting (Nations 2020). A professional network can support your career development, helping you to gain a deeper understanding of happenings within the nutrition and dietetics worldwide community.

Developing a LinkedIn profile enables you to create an online professional presence. It means when your name is put into a search engine such as Google, you will appear in the search results, which can help open doors to some opportunities. LinkedIn profiles are used to showcase your professional experience, achievements, recommendations and more. It is important to treat your LinkedIn profile in a similar way to your CV and ensure that everything that is on your profile is promoting you in the best way possible. Other professionals can recommend and endorse you for your skills and past work, which can strengthen your profile as it shows experts supporting your claims to have certain skills. LinkedIn is also a useful tool for researching organisations and the people who work at them.

Other types of social media

Social media can take many forms including: Twitter, Facebook, Instagram, WhatsApp, Slack, Clubhouse, Strava, YouTube, Vimeo, Pinterest, Snapchat, TikTok, even blogging and podcasts could be included, with more platforms being created all the time.

Social media can provide a great way to network and interact with other professionals in your field as well as being a way of sharing knowledge. Social media is open to everyone and so it can offer a way to engage with the public and raise awareness. It can also help raise the profile of Dietitians and Associate/Registered Nutritionists in general. It is a great way to publicise new research or events such as public lectures. If you are new to a particular platform, perhaps join and just watch and read for a while, then as you get more confident with how the platform works, you may want to start posting.

Remember that your posts are public and it may not be just your friends who read them. You may want to keep private and professional aspects of your life separate, so do check the privacy settings for each particular platform as you may be able to limit who sees your posts, or only allow followers you approve. Remember to check the geolocator on your account and posts; this is a safety issue as you could inadvertently be giving someone information about where you live.

Think before posting: complaints will be seen by others and so social media is not the place to air any grievances. Never drink alcohol and post! You also need to ensure you do not breach any confidentiality agreements, so you must never post pictures of patients or clients unless you have permission, nor give information that could be used to identify a colleague or patient.

Photos

Check your content before posting images. Photos can make your post look more interesting and get attention, but do you really want your future boss to have seen you in your swimwear? Also check you have permission to post photos of other people; you could always use stock photos instead.

Evidence-based information

Make sure your posts are well informed: don't just retweet or repost something that lots of other people have posted if you are not sure about the origin and authenticity of the information. It is best to stick to accurate evidence-based facts.

Be careful of buzz words and hashtags that are used to link posts on specific topics. These are constantly changing but one example is 'Clean eating'. This may mean different things to different people, but it has been in the past associated with orthorexia nervosa (an unhealthy obsession with healthy eating) and could be harmful. Associations have been found between social media use and eating concerns in young adults (Sidani et al. 2016). Furthermore, a recent study by Turner and Lefevre (2017) reported an online survey of 680 social media users found that more time spent on Instagram was associated with a greater tendency towards orthorexia nervosa, although the authors pointed out that they did not find this effect with other social media channels. Their findings highlighted the implications that social media can have on psychological wellbeing.

Don't give advice

When people find out you are studying nutrition, or dietetics, they often have questions for you. But just as you would not give dietary advice with no context to someone you met in the street, you should not be tempted to give advice online. Without the full clinical picture, you could be causing more harm than good. Many nutritionists and dietitians put on their profiles 'tweets do not equal advice'. If in doubt, recommend your contact gets in touch with their GP or another health professional.

Disagreements

Social media can be a great place to debate different issues and there will be times when you do not agree with someone. Debate can be healthy but ensure that you are respectful of the views of others and kind at all times. Consider: would you be better conducting the conversation offline?

Looking after your own mental health

Invariably at some point on social media you may come across trolls or people who behave inappropriately. In these cases, it is perfectly fine to block them. If you do not want to block them but you do not want to read their posts, then mute them. Inappropriate, abusive or harmful material can be reported on all platforms. Take screenshots as evidence. The Citizens Advice Bureau and the police can also provide further guidance on harassment.

It is also not a good idea to compare yourself to others on social media. Remember that most people will share their triumphs but not the things that didn't go so well; it's also easy to exaggerate or filter/crop photos in flattering ways. Be pleased for other people but don't necessarily take everything at face value.

It can also be sensible from time to time to take a break from social media. Time out can provide clarity and think about why you want to be on social media. You can go back whenever you are ready, or not at all, as the case may be.

Adverts on social media

Adverts should be indicated using one of the following hashtags: #Ad, #Advert or #Gifted.

But, of course, this raises the question whether professionals should endorse particular products. We have seen arguments that it is better that this is done by

Figure 10.1 A guide to social media (Source @AFNutr 2020)

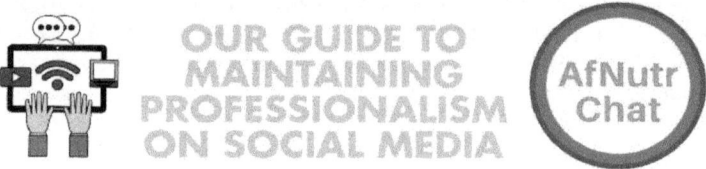

BE PROUD OF YOUR PROFESSION

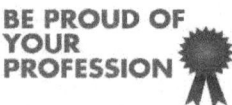

Include your AfN Registrant status in your profile description. Consistent and regular use of our titles will help individuals understand who to trust.

BE CLEAR ON WHO YOU ARE

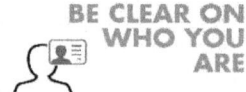

Being clear about who you are can help build trust on social media. Having a clear profile picture can help you to better connect with your audience.

KNOW YOUR LIMITS

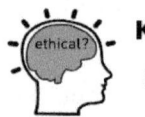

Adhere to AfN Standards of Ethics, Conduct & Performance at all times. Providing advice on an area you are not trained or competent in should be avoided.

BE POLITE AND RESPECTFUL

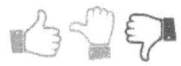

It is ok to disagree with others on social media, but be mindful of how you express this. Being rude or confrontational is unlikely to encourage scientific debate on a topic. However much you disagree - you can always be kind.

POWERFUL PICS

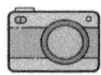

Pictures are a great way to add interest to your posts, but be mindful of any potential negative impact. Avoid posting endless streams of appearance-focussed photos, for example picture-perfect dishes or gym selfies - keep it real. Always make sure you have permission to use images, i.e., not subject to copyright. Ask for permission first.

PROMOTING PRODUCTS OR BRANDS

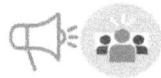

If you are involved in the promotion or advertising of products/services you must ensure that scientific knowledge, professional skills & experience are used in an accurate and responsible manner. Prominent use of #Ad #Advert or #Gifted upfront will ensure it is obvious to readers. Stay compliant with nutrition and health claims regulations, especially concerning endorsements.

BE MINDFUL OF PRIVACY

Whatever settings you choose, privacy and confidentiality can never be guaranteed on social media. As a general rule: don't say or reveal anything on social media that you wouldn't be happy to see in the press.

SUPPORT YOUR COLLEAGUES

As stated in AfN Standards of Ethics, Conduct & Performance, Registrants should be willing to share their knowledge and expertise with fellow Registrants and students. Treat others online in a way you would like to be treated.

This resource was prepared and written by AfNutr co-founders Dr Suzanne Zaremba, Dr Laura Wyness, Lynn Burns & Vicki Pyne qualified professionals rather than unqualified influencers; however there is a risk of conflict of interest. Although dietitians and registered nutritionists can play a role in the development of particular products, and research on the effects on health, it is not necessarily their role to endorse products. At all times you need to consider whether the scientific evidence is being presented in a fair and balanced way and if it is evidence based and accurate. You also need to ensure that you comply with the regulations from the Nutrition & Health Claims Regulations, Advertising Standards Authority, Competition and Markets Authority, as well as your professional body.

The infographic above (Fig. 10.1) was created by the AfNutr cofounders Dr Suzanne Zaremba, Dr Laura Wyness, Lynn Burns and Vicki Pine (2020) and summarises the best ways to remain professional on social media. Although designed with Associate and Registered Nutritionists in mind, the content equally applies to Dietitians.

Summary

As you start to look at the options beyond your degree, you will want to consider the next steps to take to start your dream career. Think about the skills, the volunteering and the work experience you have gained and how to present these on your CV and on application forms. Don't forget to check your university's careers centre for help and ideas too. You may also want to consider if social media is right for you, and ensure you maintain your professionalism online. Good luck in your chosen career.

Reflective questions

- Could you compile a CV that includes a personal profile, your academic and transferable skills, and any work and volunteering experience?
- Double check your posts and or tweets before posting. Do they sound professional and are the photos/images appropriate?
- Do you enjoy social media or is it becoming increasing stressful? If so, could you take a break?

Suggested further reading

British Dietetic Association (2021) The BDA and social media. Available at: https://www.bda.uk.com/about-us/the-bda-and-social-media.html (accessed 8 November 2021).
Moreau, E. (2020) What is a LinkedIn profile? Available at: https://www.lifewire.com/what-is-a-linkedin-profile-4587447 (accessed 5 November 2021).

References

AfNutr, Zaremba, S., Wyness, L., Burns, L. and Pine, V. (2020) Professionalism in social media. Available at: https://afnutr.wordpress.com/professionalism-on-social-media/ (accessed 5 November 2021).

Bhardwa, S. (2018) What are the benefits of student volunteering? Available at: https://www.timeshighereducation.com/student/news/what-are-benefits-student-volunteering (accessed 11 February 2021).

Lederer, A.M., Autry, D.M., Day, C.R.T. and Oswalt, S.B. (2015) The impact of work and volunteer hours on the health of undergraduate students, *Journal of American College Health*, 63(6): 403–408.

Nations, D. (2020) What is LinkedIn and why should you be on it. Available at: https://www.lifewire.com/what-is-linkedin-3486382 (accessed 3 September 2021).

Neves, J. (2018) *UK Engagement Survey.* Available at: https://www.advance-he.ac.uk/sites/default/files/2019-05/Advance_HE_UKES_2018_sector_results_report_0.pdf (accessed 8 February 2021).

Sidani, J.E., Shensa, A., Hoffman, B. et al. (2016) The association between social media use and eating concerns among US young adults, *Journal of the Academy of Nutrition and Dietetics*, 116: 1465–72. 10.1016/j.jand.2016.03.021 (accessed 5 November 2021).

Turner, P.G. and Lefevre, C.E. (2017) Instagram use is linked to increased symptoms of orthorexia nervosa, *Eating and Weight Disorders*, 22: 277–284, https://doi.org/10.1007/s40519-017-0364-2 (accessed 5 November 2021).

University of Manchester Careers Service (2021) Transferable skills. Available at: https://www.careers.manchester.ac.uk/findjobs/skills/ (accessed 2 July 2021).

11 Consultations

Overview and outline

This chapter on consultations provides you with a step-by-step guide to consultation as a nutritionist or dietitian (one-to-one or groups) and introduces you to motivational interviewing, with references to further resources for more detailed understanding of the subject.

Working as a nutritionist or a dietitian will often require you to communicate effectively with a hugely diverse range of people. A person-centred approach requires you to develop good communication skills, to enable you to develop an understanding of the needs and preferences of the individual, empowering them to make informed decisions about their lifestyle. It is rightly the case that effective communication is a required standard for registered nutritionists and dietitians in the UK (Association for Nutrition (AfN) 2021; Health and Care Professions Council (HCPC) 2021).

'The art of nutrition/dietetic practice is to integrate the science of food (and medicine) with psychosocial aspects of people's lives in the context of changing health related behaviours' (Pearson and Croker 2019).

This chapter will focus on the practical aspects of an individual consultation and the planning and delivery of group education sessions. We will only touch upon factors influencing food choice and behaviour change models as within your nutrition or dietetics degree programme you will cover these in detail; we have suggested useful resources for further reading at the end of the chapter. We aim to introduce you to planning group education sessions and individual consultations, and considerations needed for informal advice for friends and family, as well as formal aspects of private practice.

The AfN and HCPC standards of ethics, conduct and performance must be upheld at all times by ANutr, RNutr and RDs respectively; we have selected those that link directly to consultations and group education sessions below. It is important to be aware 'an ANutr will normally be working with relevant professional oversight, supervised and/or mentored. An ANutr will not normally engage in wholly independent practice' (Association for Nutrition 2021). For further understanding of the AfN and HCPC standards read chapters 12 and 13.

Table 11.1 Standards for Associate Registered Nutritionist and Registered Dietitians

AfN standards	HCPC standards
• Act in the best interest in clients,	• Promote and protect the interest of service users and carers
• Work within his/her scope of practice,	• Work within the limits of your knowledge and skills
• Maintain client confidentiality,	• Respect confidentiality
• Maintain accurate client records including informed consent,	• Keep records of your work
• Communicate effectively with clients	• Communicate appropriately and effectively
• Hold appropriate indemnity provision	

(*Source*: Table based on information from AfN 2021; HCPC 2021).

Figure 11.1 COM-B model of behaviour change (modified from Michie et al. 2011)

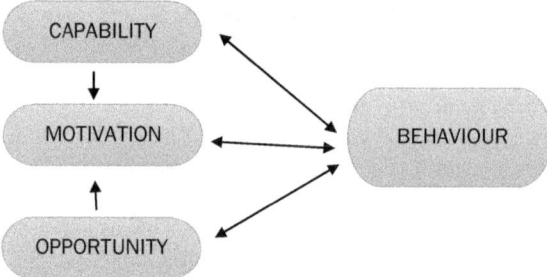

Changing behavior

The COM-B model of behaviour change includes three components to any behaviour: capability, opportunity and motivation. In order to perform a particular behaviour, a person must feel they are both psychologically and physically able to do so (capability), have the social and physical opportunity for the behaviour (opportunity), and want or need to carry out the behaviour more than other competing behaviours (motivation).

As each of these components interact, individual and group dietary interventions need to target the capability, motivation and/or opportunity in order to enable effective and sustainable behaviour change (Michie et al. 2011). We have included the COM-B model of behaviour change to remind you of its importance when considering how you conduct individual consultations or plan and deliver group education sessions.

Language you use (verbal, written and non-verbal)

The language used by nutritionists and dietitians can have a profound impact on how people feel. Inclusive and values-based language can lower anxiety, build confidence, educate and help to improve self-care. On the other hand, poor communication can be stigmatising, hurtful and undermining of self-care and also have a detrimental effect on clinical outcomes. By reflecting and increasing your awareness of your own unconscious or conscious biases you can improve your ability to communicate effectively.

For example:

> *'Being described as "non-compliant" is awful and does not reflect the fact that everyone is doing their best, maybe not the same best as someone else, or even their best "best" but just the best they can at that moment. Life is way more than Type 1 Diabetes and it isn't always given top priority. Life gets in the way.'*
> (Person with Type 1 diabetes)

An example of this is the increasingly well-documented weight bias, defined as negative attitudes towards, and beliefs about, others because of their weight. These negative attitudes are manifested by stereotypes and/or prejudice towards people with overweight and obesity. Individuals with obesity experience stigma from educators, employers, health professionals, the media, friends and family. Reflect on your attitude and those around you to weight.

For further reading see the excellent NHS England (2018) document *Language Matters*, and Language Matters: Obesity (2020) details in the Suggested further reading section at the end of this chapter.

Step-by-step guide for one-to-one consultations

As a student nutritionist or dietitian, you are likely to come across the following scenario whereby a friend or relative asks for advice; *'You're studying nutrition, could you give me a diet plan so I can lose weight?'* We are confident that through your degree you will be knowledgeable in the latest evidence for different approaches to weight loss and behaviour change models; the question here is *how* will you turn your knowledge into practical advice for others and *how* can you help others to change their behaviour?

Reflect on how you would respond to this request by a friend or relative, and how confident you would be in your approach. In this section we will provide you with a step-by-step approach to help you develop your one-to-one consultation skills. The guidance here is suitable for more formal face-to-face, telephone and online video one-to-one consultations; it is also important to consider many of these factors for informal conversations. This step-by-step guide is generic and will need to be adapted to individual situations/dietary conditions. Our aim is to give you a sound starting point.

Preparation before any consultation can begin

First, consider is the request within your area of competency? This will vary greatly on where you are in your degree, training and prior experience. Only proceed if you are competent; you should discuss with a colleague or a supervisor/mentor if you are unsure.

Before starting a consultation, check you have the relevant background information. This may take many different approaches but essentially you will need to know if the person has any medical conditions that could influence your consultation. In private practice this information can be gathered through a form that clients are required to complete before the consultation is scheduled; this will also help to inform you if you are working within your scope of practice. It is up to you to find out as the client may not be aware of its relevance; for example, you should be aware if the client has any medical condition that may influence dietary advice, such as Type 1 diabetes.

Example of pre-consultation questions that could be included:

a Current diagnoses and/or medical problems
b Past medical problems
c Current medications
d Are you awaiting any medical tests, results or operations? Give details.
e Are there any social or psychological issues I should know about, e.g. recent traumas or upheavals?
f Known food allergies/intolerances
g Foods or drinks you avoid

Consider the environment for a consultation

Consider the environment you will be working in whether that is the physical space or the background noise/visuals on a computer screen. For the physical space, are the desk and chairs set up as you would wish, having a desk between you and your client/patient is seen as an obstacle to communication, a better way would be to sit diagonally as illustrated below.

Consider the temperature of the room and whether direct sunlight will be in the eyes of either of you; you are aiming to create an environment in which neither of you are distracted by your surroundings. For online video consultations, consider your background and ensure it is professional or, if not possible, use a suitable virtual background available within video conferencing software. Consider possible noise and interruptions and put in a plan to minimise these.

Figure 11.2 The working environment for consultations considering desk, chairs and computer placement

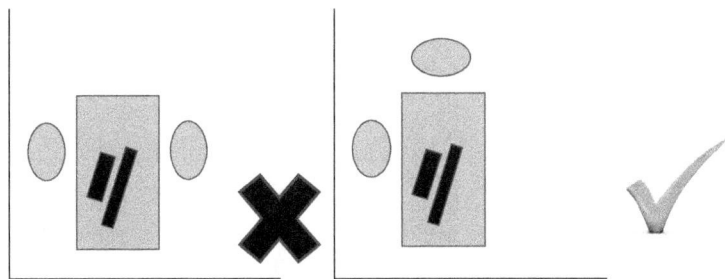

The consultation: meeting and greeting

The first few moments of a consultation are very important: this is when people form their first impressions and these can be hard to shift once formed. Aim to smile and speak in a warm tone to initiate a welcoming and friendly start to the consultation. You would usually introduce yourself and check you have the correct details and pronunciation of the client's name. Ask what the client would like to be called, including their title, e.g. Ms, Mrs etc. You can include some small talk, such as about the weather or travel, to help the client feel more at ease. It is useful to state the time available for the consultation and what will happen during the consultation. For example, 'We have 45 minutes available today, so we'll start with you explaining your condition and how it affects you, then I will ask some questions and then we can discuss potential ways forward.' If you need measurements, such as body weight or height, it is useful to mention these at the start too.

Figure 11.3 Suggested framework for an individual consultation (Pearson and Croker 2019)

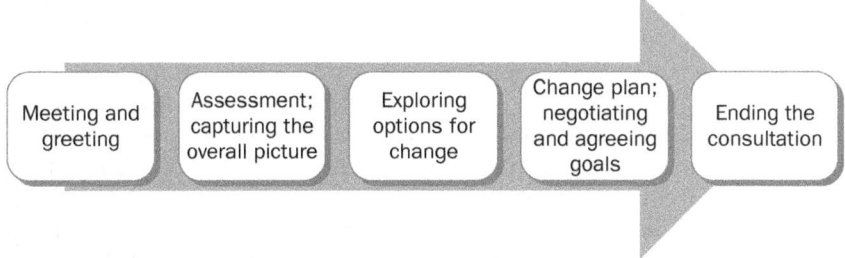

The consultation: assessment, capturing the overall picture

The client should be given the opportunity to describe their perspective; this can be achieved by using open questions to identify the issues which the individual wishes to address. For example, 'If we could start with you explaining in your words why you are here and what you hope to be addressed/achieved.' You need to listen attentively, allowing the client to complete statements without being interrupted and leaving space for them to think. This will help you to gain an understanding not just of what is happening, but how it is affecting them (including occupation and/or interests etc.).

Table 11.2 Useful communication skills

Communication skill	Example of skill
Positive non-verbal communication	Eye contact, smiling, nodding, open posture
Use verbal encouragers	'uh huh, mm, go on'
Open questions	'Would you like to tell me a bit more about that?"
Paraphrasing	You give the essence of what has been said in your own words to show your understanding of what the client has said
Establish clarity	'Could you explain to me how that affects you?'
Reflect on what is said and from non-verbal communication	'You seem quite concerned about that'
Summarise – including the content and feelings to check you have the key information about the situation	'Is there anything else you would like to add? Have I understood that right?'

(adapted from DietComms 2021)

It is important to check that the client feels confident about their knowledge of the condition, if relevant. If further information is needed, provide a clear and concise lay person's language explanation – avoiding jargon. You should then check if that information has been helpful or if more is needed.

To collect relevant anthropometric and dietary information you should explain why the information is needed and indicate that there are quite a lot of questions coming; ask permission, for example 'Is that okay with you?' and 'Would you mind if I take some notes so that I have a record of what you have told me?' The information needed will vary depending on the client's needs: you may require a detailed weight history covering several years, alternatively this may be less relevant and recent weight gain/loss is more appropriate.

Blood results, scans and other medical information are relevant for certain medical conditions; this could be information you collate before the consultation.

Asking a person to reveal what they eat can feel very personal. This needs to be considered and starting with an open question can often elicit a lot of information. For example, 'Could you tell me how food fits into your day?' will often obtain information about the context of the food intake as well as the actual foods eaten. A non-judgemental approach to eating habits is essential; you are aiming to develop a rapport with the client and help them to achieve their goals.

Exploring options for change together

Some explanation of the principles of the diet in question is likely to be required, perhaps by going through a diet sheet or using other visual aids, for example the Department of Health Eatwell guide.

It is crucial to establish a good understanding of the client's history as they may have tried to control their diet in some way for years; this is where collecting the relevant information earlier in the consultation is valuable. Be vigilant for disordered eating behaviours and show respect for your client's knowledge, experiences and efforts.

Ideally the client should be encouraged to come up with their own ideas that they consider achievable. It can be very easy for a dietitian or nutritionist to see lots of ways that a client could improve their diet and lifestyle as they complete the assessment. However, it is important to keep a person-centred approach and work with the changes the client feels they can make. People are more likely to succeed if they select the behaviour and a target which they judge is suited to their circumstances. For example, you might say 'We could talk about change in your diet or getting more active. What do you think or would you prefer to talk about something else?'

If the client is finding it difficult, the dietitian/nutritionist can offer, for example, 'Would you like me to make some suggestions/recommendations?' You should give the client an opportunity to say if anything is not likely to work for them; for example, 'Do you think this is something that you would be able to achieve?'

Activity

A person works long hours in a sedentary job and has a busy family life. He is overweight with high blood pressure.
  Using the COM-B model:

- What do you think about their psychologically and physically capability to change?
- What do you think about their social and physical opportunity to change?
- What do you think about possible motivation for change?

Some people may not be ready to make changes and feel that they do not have adequate time to commit to making changes; for example, they could be going through a particularly busy or stressful time in their work or personal life. As part of your course, you may have come across the Prochaska and DiClemente's trans-theoretical model of change (1984).

Figure 11.4 A theoretical model of change (Prochaska and DiClemente 1984)

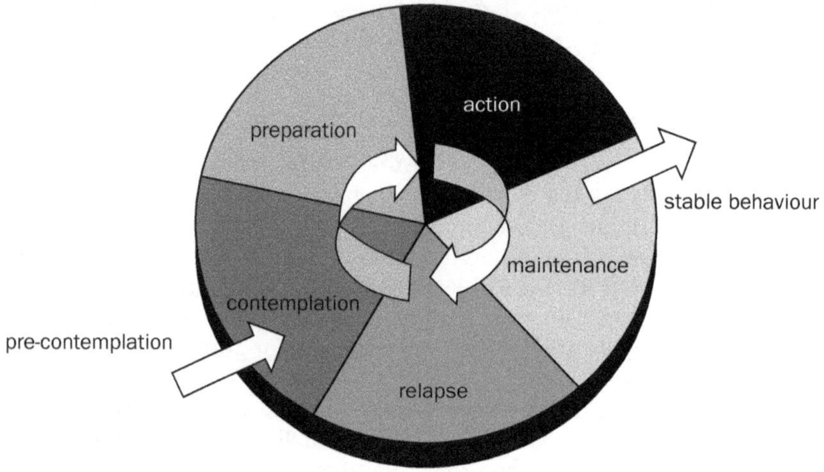

stages of change model

Here, the best approach may be to have a discussion towards getting ready for change – helping the client move from pre-contemplation to contemplation is a valuable intervention. Consider 'What is holding this person back from changing their diet?'

You should not underestimate the sustained effort required to make behavioural changes and the social and family influences that contribute to behaviour change. You could clarify that changes can be made in 'small steps' rather than 'substantial leaps' to be more achievable and sustained within the important aspects of their lifestyle.

You could start a conversation about the value of making changes that is relevant to the person and which they can relate to; for example, 'What benefits would you like to get from?' less processed foods.

Change plan: negotiating and agreeing goals

Once a person has made the decision to change, a change plan can be constructed with the help of the practitioner; see example below (figure 11.5). It is often wise that only a small number of goals are set initially (maybe three or four). Consider using SMART goals:

Specific: It could be an amount of time doing a specific behaviour, e.g. 'For the month of July, I will walk 10,000 steps a day'. It's good to reinforce positive achievements rather than have an unachievable plan; once achieved another goal can be set.

Measurable: For example, 10,000 steps a day for one month.

Achievable: The agreed goal needs to be achievable; aim to break up weight loss goals into smaller chunks that are more achievable.

Relevant: Consider how you plan to achieve the goal, discuss when extra walking can be included into the day and discuss likely barriers that may make it difficult.

Time-bound: For one month, once achieved, the goal can be reviewed by the client and they could aim to keep the 10,000 steps a day for another month, then once achieved set another goal. It may be that 10,000 steps a day is not achievable for the long term but the client realises that doing 8,000 steps is regularly possible and this could be substantially more than the client's starting point.

Figure 11.5 An example change plan

The reason(s) I am planning to change are...
Examples: to feel better, to be healthier, to be active with family without getting out of breath...

If I don't change I may...
Examples: develop more health issues/worsen those already experiencing

I am planning to ...
Examples: become more active, eat more fruit and vegetables

I am going to achieve this by...
Include Specific, Measurable, Achievable, Relevant and Time-Bound (SMART) goals

People who will help me...
Example: ask my partner not to eat snacks in front of me.

Difficulties I expect to occur are...and ideas to overcome these
Example: feeling hungry and tired; plan what I want to eat beforehand so that I know I can't have the extra nibbles.

Reward(s) to help me...
Example: Set aside time for relaxing/hobby

Ending the consultation

Whilst you will have made goals collaboratively with the client, it is important to summarise them (or ask the client to) to ensure that the client understands the goals and feels that they are achievable.

It is often useful to write a clear and succinct action plan of what has been agreed and when they intend to start. If several goals have been agreed, it is helpful to come to an agreement as to which goals to prioritise.

Agree the next steps and what options are available to them; for example when they will have another appointment and how this will be arranged. Will they be able to contact you directly, for example have a telephone call in between face-to-face appointments? This can also be a good time to evaluate how the client feels about the consultation and how confident they are about making the changes.

> **Important**
>
> Successful consultation will require you to maintain a non-judgemental attitude throughout, acknowledge the client's views and feelings and use appropriate non-verbal behaviour throughout the consultation.

Motivational interviewing

This is a widely acknowledged approach which uses a 'guiding style to engage clients, clarify their strengths and aspirations, evoke their own motivations for change and promote autonomy in decision making' (Rollnick 2008).

Motivational interviewing takes into account the following points:

- How we speak to people is likely to be just as important as what we say.
- Being listened to and understood is an important part of the process of change.
- The person who has the problem is the person who has the answer to solving it.
- People only change their behaviour when they feel ready – not when they are told to do so.
- The solutions that people find for themselves are the most enduring and effective.

Further resources can be found at the end of this chapter

Step-by-step group education sessions

As a nutritionist or dietitian, it is likely that you will have the opportunity to deliver group education sessions for different population groups, for example a healthy eating session for primary school children. Group education and peer support programmes aim to help people learn how to manage their own lifestyle for their health needs.

We are confident that through your degree you will have the appropriate knowledge and know where to source information and determine the quality of that information to put a presentation together; the question here is *how* will you turn your knowledge into practical advice for others and *how* can you help others to change their behaviour?

> **Remember**
>
> Information provision alone is unlikely to be sufficient to motivate sustainable behaviour change.

This step-by-step guide is generic; it will need to be adapted to different population groups and dietary conditions. Our aim is to give you a sound starting point.

Preparation before a group education session

First, consider whether the request is within your area of competency. Only proceed if you are competent; you should discuss with a colleague or a supervisor/mentor if you are unsure.

If the group session is an in-person event, you will need to consider many factors such as:

- Is it accessible to all your participants, for example if there are steps is there a ramp or lift access?
- Are there toilet facilities for everyone?
- Is there appropriate public transport and car parking if needed?
- Are there facilities for refreshments at the venue or nearby?
- For the session, is the room of suitable size, with appropriate furniture and teaching resources?
- If food preparation is required (e.g. a cooking skills session) are the kitchen facilities adequate?
- What is the cost of the venue hire?

Once the venue has been confirmed, consider signage to enable your participants to find the room and facilities and feel welcomed when they arrive.

If the group session is an online event, do your participants have access to the required technology and sufficient broadband to allow for seamless online video streaming?

The timing of the sessions must be given careful consideration to the participants' lifestyle and needs, for example an evening or weekend may work well for working adults to minimise time off work; whereas full-time parents may need to find childcare cover in an evening and prefer sessions during school hours.

What content to include

A good place to start is to give consideration to your audience/participants/patients: what do you think they will already know/be able to do?

What are your aims for the session(s)? For example, what are you aiming for them to know and be able to do after attending your session(s)? This will involve developing some learning outcomes. These can help to make it clear what benefits the participants can expect from attending a session(s); for example, 'at the end of this cooking session participants will have more confidence to shop and prepare a meal from raw ingredients'.

SMART goals can also be used for group sessions.

Specific: 'At the end of this sessions participants will be able to use food labels to identify foods, outside of the "free from" supermarket aisle, that are gluten free'.

Measurable: Often this is knowledge, confidence or skills. For the example above it could be, 'identify five foods' they would be likely to eat.

Achievable: Be realistic in what can be achieved within the time available.

Relevant: The goal needs to be relevant to the individuals; in our example do not specify the types of food – let the participants decide on the gluten-free foods they would usually eat, this makes it of greater relevance to their life-style.

Time bound: For example, by the end of the session. It could be a task for people to try between sessions, for example, before the next session, to identify two new gluten-free foods.

How to deliver the session

A good start is writing a lesson plan, acknowledging what will be covered, when and by who. During your degree you will develop the knowledge of what to include within a group education session.

Consider the following points when designing your content:

- Use inclusive messages and avoid those that stigmatise individuals.
- Tailor your information and activities to be relevant to the people attending.
- Use clear, simple language and avoid medical/nutrition jargon.
- Where possible use foods rather than nutrients to communicate.
- Aim for positive messages (eat more fruit/vegetables), rather than negative (eat less fat).
- Emphasise the benefits of change.
- Acknowledge the barriers to change.

Peer support is an important element of group education sessions, so factor in activities and time for participants to discuss matters with each other.

Important

Successful education sessions will require you to maintain non-judgemental attitudes, acknowledge the group's views and feelings and use appropriate non-verbal behaviour throughout.

Ending the session

It is good to summarise what has been covered in the session and the goals and outcomes, highlighting where positive changes have occurred and any plans for change that have been agreed. Make it clear if the participants are able to contact you or where to go for further resources.

Specific considerations for private practice

Starting a nutrition/dietetic consultancy business is something that many nutritionists and dietitians consider; Here is a list of factors to consider and explore:

- Decide on your offering – individual consultations, sessions for companies, writing articles? What will you focus on as your area of expertise with an awareness of your level of competency, e.g. women's health, sports performance nutrition, etc.
- Marketing yourself and your business.
- Consider your online and physical presence (e.g. consulting room).
- Insurance – indemnity provision is required.
- Data protection for your client information, General Data Protection regulations (GDPR) and requirements.
- Setting fees, accounts and record keeping.
- Will you need resources, for example written information for clients?
- Find a mentor to help you fulfil your potential and guide you towards success. If you are an ANutr, this is a requirement.
- Continuing professional development and access to resources, such as full text journal articles.

Summary

Individual consultations and group education sessions are about so much more than providing information: they are opportunities to help individuals plan and self-manage their diet and lifestyle to suit their individual circumstances and needs. Whilst the nutritionist or dietitian may be an expert in nutrition and medical conditions, the client/patient is the real expert of their own life, what is important to them and what is feasible for them to change and achieve, with your guidance and support as the nutritionist or dietitian.

The chapter is just a starting point on an exciting journey of developing skills to assist diet and lifestyle behaviour change. Many nutritionists and dietitians go on to take further courses and qualifications in behaviour change to assist them in developing greater awareness and skills in this area.

Reflective questions

- Do you know the AfN or HCPC standards that relate to dietary consultations and group education sessions?
- Think about how you would respond to a friend or relative asking for dietary advice: how would you go about it?

Suggested further reading

Avery, A., Whitehead, K. and Halliday, V. (2016) *How to Facilitate Lifestyle Change: Applying Group Education in Healthcare.* Oxford: Wiley Blackwell.

Gable, J. and Herrmann, T. (2016) *Counselling Skills for Dietitians,* 3rd edn. New Jersey: Wiley Blackwell.

Hilliard, M.E., Rickett, K.A., Ockene, J.K. and Pbert. L. (2018) *The Handbook of Health Behaviour Change.* New York: Springer Publishing.

NHS England (2018) *Language Matters: Language and Diabetes.* Available at: https://www.england.nhs.uk/wp-content/uploads/2018/06/language-matters.pdf (accessed 8 November 2021).

Obesity UK (2020) Language Matters: Obesity https://static1.squarespace.com/static/5b-c74880ab1a6217704d23ca/t/5f2b2a2e8de2001581548c86/1596664441149/Obesity+Language+Matters+FINAL_Updated+ref.pdf (accessed 6 January 2022)

Royal College of Nursing (2021) How motivational interviewing works. Available at: https://www.rcn.org.uk/clinical-topics/supporting-behaviour-change/motivational-interviewing (accessed 24 June 2021).

World Health Organization (2017) *Weight Bias and Obesity Stigma: Considerations for the WHO European Region.* Available at: https://www.euro.who.int/en/health-topics/noncommunicable-diseases/obesity/publications/2017/weight-bias-and-obesity-stigma-considerations-for-the-who-european-region-2017 (accessed 24 June 2021).

There are many CPD opportunities and postgraduate courses that also focus on behaviour change so look out for them too.

References

Association for Nutrition (2021) Association for Nutrition (AfN). Available at: https://www.associationfornutrition.org (accessed 24 June 2021).

DietComms (2021) *DietComms.* Available at: https://www.nottingham.ac.uk/dietcomms/ (accessed 24 June 2021).

Health and Care Professions Council (2021) *The Standards of Proficiency for Dietitians.* Available at: https://www.hcpc-uk.org/standards/standards-of-proficiency/dietitians/ (accessed 26 January 2021).

Michie, S., van Stralen, M.M. and West, R (2011). The behaviour change wheel: a new method for characterising and designing behaviour change interventions, *Implementation Science* 6: 42, doi:10.1186/1748-5908-6-42 (accessed 8 November 2021).

Pearson, D. and Croker, H. (2019) Chapter 1.3 Changing health behaviour, in J. Gandy (ed.) *The Manual of Dietetic Practice,* 6th edn. Oxford: Wiley Blackwell.

Prochaska, J.O. and DiClemente, C.C. (1984) *The Transtheoretical Approach: Crossing Traditional Boundaries of Therapy.* Homewood, IL: Dow Jones Irwin.

Rollnick, S. (2008) *Motivational Interviewing in Health Care.* London: The Guildford Press.

Webster-Gandy, J., Madden, A. and Holdsworth, M. (eds) (2020) *Oxford Handbook of Nutrition and Dietetics,* 3rd edn. Oxford: Oxford University Press.

12 Being a Registered Nutritionist

Overview and outline

Many of you are studying Nutrition at university in order to become an Associate Registered Nutritionist with the aim of going on to become a Registered Nutritionist. This chapter will describe the difference between an Associate Registered Nutritionist and a Registered Nutritionist and other Nutrition professionals, as well as outlining their scopes of practice. There will also be an introduction to the membership organisation, the Association for Nutrition, its code of conduct and ethics statements, and highlight essentially what it means to be a Registered Nutritionist.

What is a Registered Nutritionist?

Nutritionists are experts in the field of diet, food and health. They have in-depth knowledge about the effects of diet on health and keep up with all the latest research in this area. However, the title 'Nutritionist' is currently not protected by law. This means that essentially anyone can call themselves a nutritionist, whether that is someone who has done a weekend course or a person who has a degree, a master's qualification or a PhD in nutrition. Because it can be challenging to work out those who are qualified to practise, and those who might be giving out potentially dangerous advice, it was decided that there needed to be a way of distinguishing those who had appropriate qualifications and experience in order to protect the public (Cade et al. 2012). For this reason, the Nutrition Society in the UK made the decision to establish a publicly available register of appropriately qualified Nutritionists who practised scientifically grounded evidence-based nutrition; this became the UK Voluntary Register of Nutritionists (UKVRN) (Buss 1998). As this part of the Nutrition Society grew, and the register became more established, it was decided to set up a separate registered charity called the Association for Nutrition (AfN 2021) which would hold the register and be an independent regulator for all Registered Nutritionists. The AfN was founded in 2010 and is governed by a Council of Charity Trustees and Directors.

One of the main aims of the AfN is to protect and benefit the public by ensuring registrants meet high standards of competence and work in a professional manner. The AfN also offers and supports relevant training by accrediting suitable programmes and giving continuing professional development (CPD) endorsement to appropriate courses.

There are three titles that are registered with the AfN:

*   Registered Associate Nutritionist (ANutr)
*   Registered Nutritionist (RNutr)
*   Fellow of the AfN (FAfN)

Registered Associate Nutritionist: Students who complete an undergraduate or postgraduate degree accredited with the AFN can be listed as a Registered Associate Nutritionist (ANutr). This acknowledges their qualification in nutrition but reflects that they may not yet have much practical experience. ANutrs can work in many settings, including academic, healthcare, the community, the food industry or the voluntary sector, for example. As a new graduate, it would be best practice to work as part of a team or be supervised by someone with more experience.

Registered Nutritionist: With three years of relevant experience and a portfolio of evidence it is then possible to graduate from ANutr to fully register as a Registered Nutritionist (RNutr). RNutrs may choose to have specialisms in animal nutrition, clinical science, food science, the food industry, media, nutrition science, public health or sport and exercise. They may work with individuals or populations, communities or the voluntary sector; they may even have international roles and work at very senior levels.

Fellow of the AfN: This is a title for those who have been an RNutr for at least five years and have made a significant contribution or advancement to the field of nutrition.

All registrants have a key role to play in improving the health of the nation and preventing diet-related non-communicable disease through assessment and promotion of balanced dietary advice that is based on scientific evidence as well as combatting misinformation. ANutr, RNutr and FAfNs need to ensure they work within their limits and their competency, have appropriate supervision and know when to refer to other professionals. It is important that any advice or recommendations are evidence based. Registrants must also ensure they follow The UKVRN Standards of Ethics, Conduct and Performance as shown in Table 12.1 and have knowledge of and keep updated the competencies that are outlined in Table 12.2.

Core competencies in nutrition

The five core competencies in nutrition outlined in Table 12.2 must be covered and then kept updated by all registrants through demonstration of knowledge and understanding for ANutrs and through demonstration of knowledge, understanding and practical application for RNutrs.

Table 12.1 The UKVRN Standards of Ethics, Conduct and Performance

Registrants must:

1. Prioritise Public Benefit

2. Practice Safely and Effectively

3. Work Within Own Limits

4. Communicate Appropriately

5. Be Honest And Trustworthy

6. Speak Up About Concerns

7. Respect And Maintain Confidentiality

8. Promote Professionalism

For full details see: https://www.associationfornutrition.org/wp-content/uploads/2021/11/ 2021-AfN-Standards-of-Ethics-Conduct-and-Performance-Approved.pdf

In order to get registration, you need to show evidence of knowledge of the core competencies. Then following registration, CPD is required and the CPD should include a range of activities that cover all five of the core competency areas over a 3-year period. If you are studying an AfN accredited degree or master's programme then the syllabus will have been checked to ensure it covers all of the competencies listed in adequate detail.

What does having an accredited degree mean?

Many nutrition degrees in the UK, both undergraduate and postgraduate, are accredited by the AfN. This means that the programme and syllabus have been approved by the AfN as covering all the competencies and ethical considerations to the standard required. In order to receive accreditation, your university lecturers probably spent a great deal of time documenting the programme, the facilities and explaining how they will ensure all the requirements will be met. This means that when you graduate you can be fast tracked to apply to be a Registered Associate Nutritionist. If you are not sure if this applies to your programme of study, you can check to see if your degree in nutrition is listed as being accredited on the AfN website: https://www.associationfornutrition.org/.

Difference between a Registered Nutritionist, a Nutritional Therapist and a Dietitian

A Registered Nutritionist, as you know from reading this chapter, is educated to at least degree level, can demonstrate evidence-based practice and is listed on the UK Voluntary Register of Nutritionists (UKVRN).

Table 12.2 Nutrition Core Competencies

Core Competency 1 – Science Knowledge and understanding of the scientific basis of nutrition. Understanding nutritional requirements from the molecular through to the population level – for either human or animal systems.

Core Competency 2 – Food or Feed Chain Knowledge and understanding of the food or feed chain and its impact on food or feed choice. Integrating the food or feed supply with dietary intake for either human or animal systems.

Core Competency 3 – Social/Behaviour Knowledge and understanding of food or feed in a social or behavioural context, at all stages of the life course.

Core Competency 4 – Health/Wellbeing – Understanding how to apply the scientific principles of nutrition for the promotion of health and wellbeing of individuals, groups and populations; recognising benefits and risks.

Core Competency 5 – Professional Conduct – Understanding of professional conduct and the Association for Nutrition's Code of Ethics with evidence of good character.

Source: https://www.associationfornutrition.org/wp-content/uploads/2020/06/COMPETEN-CY-REQUIREMENTS-FOR-REGISTERED-NUTRITIONIST-REGISTRATION-2019.pdf

Nutritional Therapists may have different qualifications and voluntary registration is with the Complementary and Natural Healthcare Council (CNHC 2021) which registers complementary health practitioners.

The title Registered Dietitian is protected by law for those registered with the Health and Care Professions Council (HCPC 2021). Dietitians are qualified to work in the NHS or in the community, with both healthy and sick individuals as well as the wider public. The role of dietitians will be discussed in more detail in the next chapter.

Nutrition Society

Many Registered Nutritionists and Dietitians are also members of the Nutrition Society. This is an academic and learned society, first set up in 1941, and as mentioned earlier it was instrumental in the establishment of the AfN. Its aims are to advance the scientific study of nutrition and the application of this knowledge. The Nutrition Society organises conferences, training and publishes academic journals with the latest scientific research. It also offers some awards and grants, including the student vacation bursary and travel grants for members. As well as full membership there are student and recent graduate membership options available. The Society also provides further opportunities to network with other Nutrition and Dietetic professionals.

Sport and Exercise Nutrition Register

The Sport and Exercise Nutrition Register (SENR) is another voluntary register that provides accreditation for those who are appropriately qualified and experienced enough to work independently in the area of sport and exercise and directly with athletes specifically. This register includes Registered Nutritionists, Dietitians and also Sport and Exercise Scientists.

Academy of Nutrition Sciences

You may also have heard of the Academy of Nutrition Sciences which has been described as 'a collective voice for evidence-based nutrition science' (Academy of Nutrition Sciences 2021). This was established in 2019 between the AfN, the British Dietetic Association, the British Nutrition Foundation and the Nutrition Society. It has essentially been set up to combine forces to champion nutrition science, to advance knowledge, support education and research, ensuring all applications of nutrition science are evidence based, to ultimately improve public health and wellbeing.

Summary

You should now have a greater understanding of what it is to be an Associate Registered Nutritionist or a Registered Nutritionist. Through understanding the core competencies and the ethics, conduct and performance expectations, it is clear there is a high level of professionalism expected of people using these titles. You may now also understand the professional relationship with other similar societies. On graduation, do consider becoming registered with the AfN and be proud of your professional status and title.

Reflective questions

- Are you aware of the UKVRN Standards of Ethics, Conduct and Performance?
- Does the knowledge you have gained so far encompass the core competencies that must be covered in order to be an Associate Nutritionist or a Registered Nutritionist?

Suggested further reading

Association for Nutrition: https://www.associationfornutrition.org/
Nutrition Society: https://www.nutritionsociety.org/
Sport and Exercise Nutrition Register: http://www.senr.org.uk/

References

Academy of Nutrition Sciences (2021) available at: https://www.academynutrition-sciences.org.uk/ (accessed 2 March 2021).

Association for Nutrition (2021) AfN. Available at: https://www.associationfornutrition. org/ (accessed 2 March 2021).

Buss, D. (1998) Registered Public Health Nutritionist (RPHNutr): a new qualification in public health nutrition, *Nutrition & Food Science*, 98: 158–62.

Cade, J., Eccles, E., Hartwell, H. et al. (2012) The making of a nutrition professional: the Association for Nutrition register, *Public Health Nutrition*, 15: 2012–19.

Complementary and Natural Healthcare Council (2021) available at: https://www.cnhc. org.uk/ (accessed 2 March 2021).

Health and Care Professions Council (2021) available at: https://www.hcpc-uk.org/ (accessed 2 March 2021).

13 Being a Dietitian

Overview

Dietetics is an exciting and dynamic career, in which knowledge and practice can change rapidly. It is an evidence-based profession with research, reflective practice and systematic clinical reasoning as fundamental principles. Having a clear understanding of your requirements from the professional regulator, the Health and Care Professions Council (HCPC), is essential. An awareness of the resources and guidance available from the professional body for dietetics, the British Dietetic Association (BDA), will assist you in your career, providing opportunities for you to develop as a dietitian. In the UK, 'dietitian' and 'dietician' are protected titles by law, and dietitians must be registered with the HCPC to use these titles. The term 'dietitian' is predominantly used in the UK. To qualify as a dietitian, you are required to undertake a university degree approved by the HCPC.

> 'A dietitian uses the science of nutrition to create eating plans for patients to treat medical conditions. They promote good health by helping to facilitate a positive change in food choices.' (HCPC 2021)
> 'Dietitians interpret the science of nutrition to improve health and treat diseases/conditions by educating and giving practical, personalised advice to clients, patients, carers and colleagues.' (BDA 2021)

An introduction to the Health and Care Professions Council (HCPC)

In order to practise as a dietitian in the UK you must be registered with the Health and Care Professions Council (HCPC). The HCPC protects the public by regulating 15 health and care professions in the UK. The Council's remit includes:

- Setting standards for professionals' education, training and practice; explaining what is expected of registered professionals.
- Approving programmes which professionals must complete in order to register with the HCPC.
- Keeping a register of professionals who meet the HCPC standards; and taking action if professionals on the Register do not meet HCPC standards.

The HCPC Standards of conduct, performance and ethics document sets out how the HCPC expects registrants to behave and what the public can expect from their health and care professional. The HCPC Standards state that dietitians must:

1 Promote and protect the interests of service users and carers
2 Communicate appropriately and effectively
3 Work within the limits of their knowledge and skills
4 Delegate appropriately
5 Respect confidentiality
6 Manage risk
7 Report concerns about safety
8 Be open when things go wrong
9 Be honest and trustworthy
10 Keep records of their work

It is important, as a student dietitian, to take the time to read and understand each of these standards (see details of the HCPC website in the further reading section at the end of this chapter). Each standard is elaborated; for example standard 1, includes "*1.5 You must not discriminate against service users, carers or colleagues by allowing your personal views to affect your professional relationships or the care, treatment or other services that you provide.*"

Activity

Go to the HCPC website, find the standards of conduct, performance and ethics. Then think of an example of how you meet each HCPC standard from examples both within your university degree and in life outside your course. For example. "Standard 2.7 You must use all forms of communication appropriately and responsibly, including social media and networking websites." When I post nutrition and diet related information on social media I am mindful that the information is evidence-based.

Alongside the HCPC standards of conduct, performance and ethics, there are the HCPC standards of proficiency; these set out the necessary standards to protect the public, indicating clear expectations of dietitians' knowledge and abilities. An approved university degree programme for dietetics will equip student dietitians to meet the standards of proficiency and register with the HCPC. The HCPC standards of proficiency state that dietitians must:

1 Be able to practise safely and effectively within their scope of practice
2 Be able to practise within the legal and ethical boundaries of their profession
3 Be able to maintain fitness to practise

4 Be able to practise as an autonomous professional, exercising their own professional judgement

5 Be aware of the impact of culture, equality and diversity on practice

6 Be able to practise in a non-discriminatory and inclusive manner

7 Understand the importance of and be able to maintain confidentiality

8 Be able to communicate effectively

9 Be able to work appropriately with others

10 Be able to maintain records appropriately

11 Be able to reflect on and review practice

12 Be able to assure the quality of their practice

13 Understand the key concepts of the knowledge base relevant to their profession

14 Be able to draw on appropriate knowledge and skills to inform practice

15 Understand the need to establish and maintain a safe practice environment

On the website each standard is elaborated on, it is important you take the time to read and understand each of these HCPC Standards of proficiency, think of examples of where you demonstrate each standard. An example "Standard 5 be aware of the impact of culture, equality and diversity on practice " this could be demonstrated during a consultation with an awareness of the persons religious beliefs and knowledge of how this may impact the nutritional advice for example "I see in your notes it mentions you are a practising Hindu, please summarise the foods that you avoid eating" This recognises that whilst Hindus do not eat beef or beef products you have awareness that there are variations in what other foods are avoided. For further reading see Thaker & Barker (2012).

A dietitian is required to renew their HCPC registration every two years. At each renewal, dietitians are required to confirm that they continue to meet the HCPC's standards, including CPD. During each renewal the HCPC randomly select 2.5 per cent of registrants to submit their CPD profile, indicating how the registrant's CPD activities meet the standards. See Chapter 14 for more information on CPD.

The British Dietetic Association (BDA)

The British Dietetic Association (BDA), established in 1936, has over 10,000 members, inclusive of HCPC-registered dietitians, dietetic students and dietetic support staff/assistant practitioners. The BDA is a professional body that aims to inform, protect, represent and support its members. It is also a trade union representing the professional, educational, public and workplace interests of members. The BDA promotes the work of dietitians in order to raise the profile of the profession. The BDA has regional branches and specialist groups; these offer geographically local or specialism networking opportunities and events. As a student dietitian you can join any of the specialist interest groups (see Table 13.1), these groups offer current information, leadership and expertise to members interested in or specialising in a particular area.

Table 13.1 British Dietetic Association specialist groups

• Critical Care	• Older People
• Cystic Fibrosis	• Optimising Nutrition Prescribing
• Diabetes	• Oncology
• Food Allergy	• Oncology, Head and Neck specialist sub-group
• Food Service	• Paediatric
• Freelance Dietitians	• Paediatric, Autism specialist sub-group
• Gastroenterology	• Paediatric, Diabetes specialist sub-group
• HIV Care	• Paediatric, Neonatal specialist sub-group
• Maternal and Fertility	• Parenteral and Enteral Nutrition
• Mental Health	• Public Health
• Mental Health, Child & Adolescent sub-group	• Renal Nutrition
• Neurosciences	• Sports Nutrition
• Obesity	• Sustainable Diets

Scope of practice

The scope of practice encompasses an impressively broad range of roles and activities within which dietitians perform. Client groups include premature babies, infants, children and all in-between up to the elderly, healthcare professionals, the public, companies, charities and the media. The majority of dietitians are involved in prevention, whether that is preventing illness developing in a healthy person/population or specific advice and guidance for a patient population to prevent complications, for example, obesity, diabetes, liver failure or dementia, to optimise their nutrition so that they can experience relief from symptoms, prevent complications and enhance their quality of life. Research and audit are integral throughout a dietitian's work and career for improving the evidence base, utilising and building upon the skills developed during your degree.

Potential careers

You may only be aware of hospital-based dietitians, and indeed a large proportion of dietitians do work within private and National Health Service (NHS)

hospitals; this is alongside dietitians who work in the community – visiting people in their homes or nursing homes – and also many advanced practice dietitians who are based in GP surgeries.

Dietitians can, and do, work in many different locations and sectors. The list is extensive but includes: public health, university teaching and research, food industry, for example companies offering specialist nutrition products (e.g. oral nutritional supplements and enteral feeds), food catering businesses, charities (e.g. Diabetes UK or Coeliac UK), elite sports clubs or organisations, freelance, journalism and the media. Throughout a dietitian's career they may specialise in different areas and move between different sectors.

Within the NHS, graduate entry is a Band 5 position, with jobs being advertised through the website: www.jobs.nhs.uk. Career progression with the NHS tends to involve specialising in an area of dietetics (Band 6) and progressing to having a leading role in the specialism (Band 7). Further progression may involve managing a dietetic or therapies department or becoming an Advanced practitioner (Band 8a, 8b), with the potential for further progression into senior management roles with the NHS. The values of the NHS are fundamental to the organisation and are shown in Fig. 13.1. Read through these values and consider how you will embrace them and ensure they reflect through your practice as a student dietitian and beyond into your career.

Figure 13.1 National Health Service (NHS) Core Values (Department of Health and Social Care 2021)

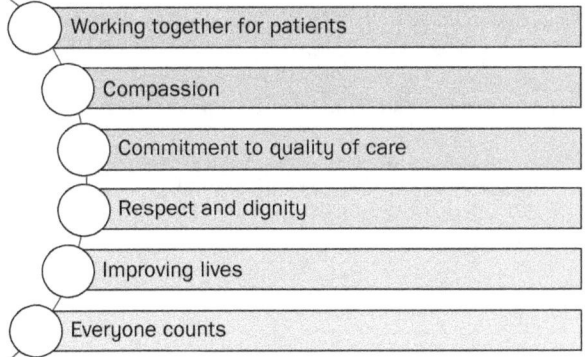

Summary

Dietetics is an evidenced-based profession requiring continual CPD to keep up to date with the new developments in research and guidance in their area of practice. To use the term 'dietitian' in the UK you need to be registered with the HCPC and abide by the standards of conduct and proficiency. Dietetics is a wide and varied career and offers many opportunities for individuals to specialise.

Reflective questions

- Are you aware of the HCPC Standards of Conduct, Performance and Ethics?
- Does the knowledge you have gained so far encompass the HCPC standards of proficiency in order to be a Registered Dietitian?

Suggested further reading

Gandy, J. (2019) *The Manual of Dietetic Practice*, 6th edn. Oxford: Wiley Blackwell.

Health and Care Professions Council (2021) *Standards of Conduct and Performance*. Available at: https://www.hcpc-uk.org/standards/standards-of-conduct-performance-and-ethics/

Health and Care Professions Council (2021) *Standards of Proficiency*. Available at: https://www.hcpc-uk.org/standards/standards-of-proficiency/dietitians/

Parenteral and Enteral Nutrition Group (2021) *Dietetic Outcomes Toolkit*. Available at: https://www.peng.org.uk/pdfs/publications/dietetic-outcomes-toolkit-updated-march-2021.pdf

Thaker, A. and Barton, A. (2012) *Multicultural Handbook of Food, Nutrition and Dietetics*. Oxford: Wiley Blackwell.

References

British Dietetic Association (2021) What do dietitians do?. Available at: https://www.bda.uk.com/about-dietetics/what-do-dietitians-do.html (accessed 28 June 2021).

Health and Care Professions Council (2021) *Standards of Proficiency*. Available at: https://www.hcpc-uk.org/standards/standards-of-proficiency/dietitians/ (accessed 28 June 2021).

Department of Health and Social Care (2021) *National Health Service (NHS) Core Values*. Available at: https://www.gov.uk/government/publications/the-nhs-constitution-for-england/the-nhs-constitution-for-england#introduction-to-the-nhs-constitution (accessed 28 June 2021).

14 CPD and staying up to date

Overview and outline

Continuing professional development (CPD) is an important way to maintain and widen your skills and knowledge. It can help you keep your knowledge and practice current, identify goals and even help you progress in your career and work towards promotions. This chapter will outline what CPD is, what it can include, the importance of keeping records of your CPD, and abiding by the requirements of the professional organisations in order to be an effective life-long learner.

What is CPD?

CPD refers to learning experiences and activities that professionals must engage in, track and document. It is important for maintaining and enhancing your skill set and for staying up to date within your profession. CPD should be considered a normal part of professional life for all professional staff (King 2015). CPD is also a requirement for registration with professional bodies such as the Association for Nutrition (AfN) and the Health and Care Professions Council (HCPC).

The learning doesn't stop when you graduate

We have found that students often see the gaining of their degree as an end point, rather than the start of their learning journey. Whilst there is much to celebrate in the achievement of this incredible milestone in your career, it does not mean the learning has to stop. On the contrary, following graduation Associate Nutritionists (ANutr), Registered Nutritionists (RNutr) and Registered Dietitians (RD) must ensure that they continue to maintain their knowledge, stay up to date to enhance and take their careers even further. In many cases it may even be required for legal and patient safety reasons. In the case of ANutrs, they need to ensure they continue their education and experience in the form of CPD to be able to progress their title to become a RNutr.

Why is CPD important?

CPD is important to maintain and extend our skills and knowledge for lifelong learning and to remain up to date as a professional. CPD does not have to be a course: it can include any activity that helps with your professional and/or personal development. It makes you responsible for your own needs and development and can increase your confidence. CPD can also be a chance to network with colleagues in a similar field; it can help you keep motivated, maintain your enthusiasm for your job and remember why you chose this career in the first place.

What counts as CPD?

There are many different activities that can count as CPD; some examples are listed here:

- Conferences
- Webinars
- Journal clubs
- Completing CPD articles in relevant magazines
- Reviewing a book
- Volunteering within the community or a school
- Twitter chats
- Peer review
- A new project
- Journal reviewer
- Writing an article or research paper
- Work-based learning
- Courses
- Peer support
- Shadowing someone
- Developing new training materials
- Further studies

Many of these activities are things that you might do without even realising they are CPD. Whatever the activity, it is important that you record it and reflect on it. Remember, from Chapter 9, that there are many theoretical models of reflection in education, but essentially reflection is simply thinking about something to make sense of it, i.e. learning from the experience. Make some notes, even bullet points, but make sure you would be able to understand those notes at some point in the future. It is also worth remembering that the recording and reflecting gets easier with practice; make it something you do regularly, perhaps once a month, so it becomes a habit.

CPD records

It is very important that you keep a record of your CPD. The professional bodies may even ask to see evidence that CPD has taken place and if your records are up to date and easily accessible this won't be an issue. Ideally, keep your records of CPD updated as you go; otherwise it is too easy to forget all the things you have done and participated in that are relevant.

You can keep organised paper files and these are particularly useful for collating your certificates. But it can be very useful to have everything in one place on a computer or at least a summary table. Excel is a good place to keep a record of your activities or you can record CPD in your account on the AfN website. We know many registrants who do both.

Your summary records should include, at least, the name of the activity, the date, the duration, any evidence and any personal reflections.

Identifying your CPD needs

Try to think about the areas that you want to develop or gaps that you need to fill. It is very easy to see a webinar or a lecture advertised and think 'that will do'. But try to plan and target for your own particular needs. You could do this by thinking about the job you are currently doing or the job that you want; perhaps you are aiming for a promotion or to progress your education. Think about this job and try to identify the knowledge and skills that you require.

Next, consider the skills you currently have. Do these skills need practice to be maintained or are you sufficiently competent in these areas and need to branch out? What do you need to achieve and maintain these skills? Is there a particular course that would help or a person who is proficient in this area that you could shadow or peer review? Do you need to spend more time reading journals on certain subject areas or would writing an article help you develop those skills further?

It is helpful to consider the time frame and plan ahead. CPD cycles are usually annual or biannual. But you might think longer term as you prepare for career progression and promotion. This is how you can focus on your current and future needs, and ensure that these needs are driven by you. You could formalise these aims in a personal development plan (PDP) and make it part of your CPD portfolio.

Personal development plans

PDPs are structures or frameworks that enable you to reflect upon your learning and achievements and then plan and set goals; essentially it means taking responsibility for your own career development (QAA 2009).

You may have come across PDPs already, at school or university, as a way of improving academic performance or starting to plan your career. You may even use them in your current job.

PDPs can help you to identify your learning and not just learning based on the curriculum as they can include personal development and extra-curricular activities and interests too.

As with any type of portfolio, PDPs can be in hard copy or online, whatever you prefer and will update as you go along.

Barriers to doing CPD

There are many reasons why people do not engage with CPD. It may be owing to lack of time, particularly if you are juggling many roles and are trying to maintain work and family balance. Look for opportunities for CPD that you may be able to complete as part of your role. Discuss with your line manager if there is any possibility of getting some time off for CPD activities. King (2015) stated that lack of personal interest and lack of encouragement are common; but find something that interests you and perhaps you could discuss with your manager or team how this may potentially improve your work and even benefit your colleagues too. Funding can also be an issue; conferences and courses can be expensive, so look out for free or subsidised places and remember that there are many free online webinars and journal clubs that are available too.

Professional societies

A recent review (Karas et al. 2020) aimed to assess how CPD compares across many different health care professions that are regulated. They found wide variation in the types of CPD being undertaken in the UK. In 81 per cent of cases, registrants needed to provide a reflection on their learning, 35 per cent were required to have a personal development plan and 26 per cent had no requirement for peer-to-peer learning. They concluded that CPD schemes vary – very much depending on the organisation. Therefore it is important that you check what your employer and professional society requires and recommends.

The Association for Nutrition and the HCPC both have their own CPD requirements and consider CPD to be essential to ensure their registrants maintain and extend their knowledge and skills, work safely and legally, build their own confidence, demonstrate commitment to their career and also, and most importantly, safeguard the public and patients.

Association for Nutrition CPD requirements

The AfN requires that all Registered Nutritionists and Associate Registered Nutritionists who have been registered for more than four years, whether they are full or part-time, should complete a minimum of 30 hours of CPD per year. The CPD should include a range of activities and furthermore, over the course of three years, the CPD activities undertaken should include all five of the core competency areas that are: Sciences, Food or Feed Chain, Social/Behaviour Knowledge, Health/Wellbeing and Professional Conduct. As 5 per cent of all Registered Nutritionists are audited each year it is important that records are kept up to date.

The AfN specifically recommended that CPD records should include:

- The date
- The activity
- The number of hours involved
- Any evidence, such as certificates
- Reflection on the activity undertaken
- Description of which core competency the CPD covered

The AfN states that CPD records can be kept in any format or even in the dedicated area on the AfN website

Guidelines for Dietitians

Dietitians in the UK are all regulated by the Health & Care Professions Council (HCPC). All HCPC registrants are required to undertake CPD and keep records of these activities.

According to the HCPC (2018) Registrants must:

1 Ensure they keep an up-to-date and continuous record of their CPD activities.
2 The CPD activities should be a mixture of activities related to current practice or aims for the future.
3 Ensure that the CPD activities have influenced the quality of their dietetic practice and service delivery.
4 Ensure that their CPD activities benefit service users.

Every other year, when registration is renewed, dietitians are asked to sign to say that they are continuing to meet the HCPC's standards, including maintaining their CPD to an acceptable level. Around the renewal period, 2.5 per cent of all dietitians will be randomly selected for audit and asked to submit their CPD files and supporting evidence that should cover the previous two years; so it is worth keeping your records up to date in case you get the call.

Summary

This chapter should have helped you to realise the importance of maintaining and expanding your skill set through CPD. There are many activities that can count as CPD and it is important that you reflect and keep a record of them, whether that is in a portfolio or a PDP, a paper version or online. You will also be aware of the importance of checking the professional society's requirements for CPD to ensure you meet their standards.

Reflective questions

- Think about what skills you need to do the job you have or the job you want; which of those skills do you lack or want to develop?
- Can you identify a course, or an activity, or even a person you could shadow, that could help you develop that skill?

Suggested further reading

Association for Nutrition (n.d.) Continuing professional development (CPD). Available at: https://www.associationfornutrition.org/careers-nutrition/cpd (accessed 8 November 2021).

British Dietetic Association (n.d.) Your CPD. Available at: https://www.bda.uk.com/practice-and-education/education/your-cpd.html (accessed 8 November 2021).

The Interprofessional CPD and Lifelong Learning UK Working Group (2019) *Principles for continuing professional development and lifelong learning in health and social care*. Available at: https://www.bda.uk.com/uploads/assets/3830abb3-e267-4f5c-a93e-7c3aca843ffe/cpdjointstatement.pdf (accessed 8 November 2021).

Health and Care Professions Council continuing Professional Development (CPD) https://www.hcpc-uk.org/cpd/ (accessed 6 January 2022).

References

Association for Nutrition (2019) https://www.associationfornutrition.org/ (accessed 8 November 2021).

Health & Care Professions Council (2018) Standards of continuing professional development. Available at: https://www.hcpc-uk.org/standards/standards-of-continuing-professional-development/ (accessed 26 January 2021).

Karas, M., Sheen, N.J.L., North, R.V. et al. (2020) Continuing professional development requirements for UK health professionals: a scoping review, *BMJ Open*, 10: e032781, doi: 10.1136/bmjopen-2019-032781 (accessed 8 November 2021).

King, H. (2015) Continuing professional development in higher education: what do academics do? *Planet*, 13: 26–29.

QAA: Quality Assurance Agency for Higher Education (2009) *Personal Development Planning: Guidance for Institutional Policy and Practice in Higher Education.* Available at: https://www.qaa.ac.uk/docs/qaas/enhancement-and-development/pdp-guidance-for-institutional-policy-and-practice.pdf?sfvrsn=4145f581_8 (accessed 8 November 2021).

Index

Page numbers with 't' indicate tables.